Exercise
Personal Training
101

Exercise
Personal Training

101

Michael Chia
Patricia Wong

National Institute of Education, Singapore

World Scientific

NEW JERSEY · LONDON · SINGAPORE · BEIJING · SHANGHAI · HONG KONG · TAIPEI · CHENNAI

Published by

World Scientific Publishing Co. Pte. Ltd.

5 Toh Tuck Link, Singapore 596224

USA office: 27 Warren Street, Suite 401-402, Hackensack, NJ 07601

UK office: 57 Shelton Street, Covent Garden, London WC2H 9HE

British Library Cataloguing-in-Publication Data
A catalogue record for this book is available from the British Library.

Desk Editor: Tjan Kwang Wei

ISBN-13 978-981-4327-88-6
ISBN-10 981-4327-88-3

Printed in Singapore.

Experts' View

The two authors have an outstanding track record of publications and applied work in the area of personal training and healthy lifestyle.

The key feature of this book is to help personal trainers to empower their clients with good problem-solving and decision-making skills concerning their health and well-being. This is a much needed addition to the literature. Several text books on personal training are available, however, the content of *"Personal Training 101"* is unique in that it provides applied and practical guidelines that cover a wide range of training and program issues. The book provides a holistic approach to personal training that is much needed to create lifestyle changes.

The book covers important training issues that are made accessible to the readers through topics such as concept statements, strategies for action, technology updates, in the news, key points and technical jargon, web-resources and follow-up references. The authors base their recommendations on research in exercise science, yet the communication of important personal training principles is accessible to everyone. The ability to translate research into practice is one of the most important assets of this book.

Jean Côté, Ph.D.
Professor and Director
School of Kinesiology and Health Studies
Queen's University, Canada

Exercise Personal Training 101 offers a personal trainer a comprehensive guide to the professional practice of assisting individuals to achieve maximum health and fitness.

Authored by two individuals who are not only outstanding scholars in the field of exercise science, but have skillfully proven themselves to have the ability to translate hard scientific evidence into applied practices for all levels of exercise professionals. As one would expect from these authors, the book covers thoroughly and interestingly covers every aspect of Personal Training programmes, but in addition covers the professional topics of ethics, beliefs, client relations and programme design.

An added bonus to the book are the multiple appendices that offer clearly, compelling and complete examples that turn the ideas of the book into easily understandable and applicable professional practices. The well conceived content of contained in this book will easily move from the pages into the practice of every exercise personal trainer.

Paul G. Schempp, Ph.D.
Professor and Director
Sport Instruction Research Lab
University of Georgia
Athens, GA 30606
USA

About the Authors

Dr Michael Chia is Head Physical Education & Sports Science and Professor of Paediatric Exercise Physilogy at the National Institute of Education, Nanyang Technological University in Singapore. He was concurrently an Association of Commonwealth Universities and a Nanyang Technological University Staff Scholar for his doctoral studies in 1995-1998. He was Vice-President of the Education Research Association of Singapore and is the Vice-President of the Asian Council of Exercise and Sports Science, a BASES-accredited sports scientist (Physiology Research) and an ACSM Health and Fitness Director. He spent five years certifying Group Exercise Leaders and Health and Fitness Instructors for Singapore and the region for the ACSM and health professionals for the private sector. He is on the Editorial Boards of the International Journal of Sports Science and Coaching, Acta Kinesiologica, Sports Science, Asian Journal of Exercise and Sports Science and The Open Education Journal. He published more than 150 journal papers, book chapters, books, monographs and articles in print and on the internet and gave more than 50 keynote and invited presentations on sport, exercise, fitness and health issues in youth and adults to national and international audiences. His research expertise is in paediatric exercise physiology and health, physical education, personal training and health education. He is well-practised as a Consultant Exercise and Health Advisor and Trainer to the Senior Management Team of a multi-national corporation and served as trainer and chief examiner for the ACSM Health and Fitness Certification courses in Singapore. He is listed in the USA Marquis publication of Who's Who in Medicine and Healthcare and Engineering and Science.

Dr Patricia Wong lectures in anatomy, exercise physiology and bioenergetics, health and wellness, nutrition, growth and development, and kinanthropometry since 1996. She graduated as an International Postgraduate Research Scholar from The University of Western Australia, where she won several academic honours and prizes during her undergraduate and postgraduate years. She is active in research in areas of obesity and exercise interventions, and has developed several specific research and educational softwares. She is also an internationally accredited Anthropometrist and Instructor for the International Society for the Advancement of Kinanthropometry. She has served as a reviewer in the field of Exercise Physiology and Nutrition for the Asian Journal of Exercise and Sports Science and in Kinanthropometry for the Journal of Sports Sciences. She has developed teaching curriculum and modules serving in different capacities as a writer, editor, advisor and project director for different organisations in Singapore. Her expertise extends to educational, curriculum and professional development consultancy projects both locally and internationally, and has taught courses that address various pedagogical issues in teaching and learning.

Preface

Personal Training 101 provides a message of empowerment for personal trainers who believe in the holistic development of their clients. The book is not just about the nuts and bolts of personal training or just about exercise or nutrition. Rather, it is about the holistic development of the client, being client-centred and process-centred as this will help ensure business longevity.

The key philosophy of the book is to help personal trainers to empower their clients with good problem-solving and decision-making skills concerning their health and well-being. This is done by subscribing and internalising HELP. HELP will serve new and experienced personal trainers in good stead in a more connected and globalised clientele. HELP explained is **H**ealth is available for **E**veryone who makes **L**ifetime changes and it is **P**ersonalised.

Using HELP, personal trainers can help all clients make personal lifetime and lifestyle changes that promote health, fitness and wellness. Good personal trainers become great personal trainers when they practise HELP with their clients and help them to become better problem-solvers and decision makers rather than telling them what to do, by offering sound and scientifically-based information that is personalised and appropriate. Additionally, the authors recommend that all personal trainers take PRIDE (personal responsibility in daily effort) in their stride, for garnering and polishing up their knowledge, skills and attitude (art and science) for great personal training.

Excellent personal trainers can be lifestyle and wellness coaches who are renowned for their great listening skills and high emotional quotient. They exceed client expectations at every opportunity. You can be one of them by making a start today.

Part I (Chapters 1-4) of the book deals with generic personal training issues while Part II (Chapters 5-10) of the book deals with specific programmes issues. Special features in the book include concept statements, strategies for action, technology updates, in the news, key points, web-resources and follow-up references.

Personal Training 101 is a must-have, whether you are starting out in personal training or an experienced personal trainer.

Much appreciation and thanks are due to Scott Weng and Ellen Huang from Taipei, Taiwan, and Ho Wei Ching, Victoria Toh and Joanna Ho from Singapore, who were all excellent and gracious models in the photographs.

Dr Michael Chia and Dr Patricia Wong

Contents

List of Tables

List of Figures

Part 1

Generic Personal Training Issues

Chapter 1

Fundamental Anchors and Beliefs in Personal Training

Fundamental anchors or beliefs are important in personal training as they shape and drive values, skills and knowledge in personal training.

After completing this chapter, you will be able to:

- ❖ Understand the qualities and values that are important in personal training.
- ❖ Verbalise and practise some of these qualities on a daily basis.
- ❖ Internalise the personal training qualities.

1.1 Introduction

Personal trainers are plentiful- many with dubious qualities and practices. Can you name some of these dubious qualities and practices? A combination of appropriate academic and professional qualifications, relevant experience in the field and human factor qualities and values is a potent recipe for success and longevity in the business of personal training.

The future of personal training in Singapore is bright as many more people living in Singapore both citizens and expatriates enjoy greater leisure and a better quality of life. Increasingly, the demand for qualified personal training services will escalate.

1.2 Essential Beliefs, Values and Qualities

Beliefs are assumptions that you make about things or people and how you expect things to be. Values are demonstrated in qualities like honesty, integrity and openness. Beliefs, values and qualities can be learned and qualities that make a good personal trainer can be ingrained and practised. For example qualities such as a cheerful and positive disposition and respect for people or clients can be a winning combination as a personal trainer.

Research and expert opinion suggest that the following fundamental anchors are useful as personal trainers:

1.2.1 *A professional health practitioner*

In a connected and globalised environment, where clients are very well informed, there is a strong expectation that the personal trainer must be knowledgeable with all that is current in health, fitness and wellness. All personal trainers should have valid certifications in cardio-pulmonary Resuscitation (CPR) and First Aid at the very least and must be familiar with medical emergency procedures.

A personal trainer must be well-networked in that he/she does not act beyond his/her area of expertise and render inappropriate and unqualified advice. A good personal trainer has formal and strong relationships with medical and sport doctors, physiotherapists, dieticians, massage therapists, chiropractors, athletic trainers, and other personal trainers.

Preferably, they should have memberships and affiliations to national and international professional bodies like the Singapore Physical Education Association, the Singapore Fitness Instructors' Association, the Sports Medicine and Sports Science Association, or the National Coaches Registry of the Singapore Sports Council, the American College of Sports Medicine, the National Strength and Conditioning Association or the British Association of Sport and Exercise Science.

1.2.2 *Occupies a position of trust and responsibility*

At all times, the personal trainer must act responsibly and earn the trust of clients. He/she must be reliable and loyal and makes adjustment where necessary to match the learning style of the client. A good emotional quotient is necessary to connect with clients with a healthy balance struck between establishing rapport and getting through a workout. They must have the client's well-being as a priority. The position of trust, reliability and responsibility must be earned and should never be betrayed.

1.2.3 *An effective communicator*

He or she must be able to establish a good working rapport with clients. He/she is well-heeled in listening, is communicative and demonstrates positive empathy with clients. He/she is able to communicate well with a wide spectrum of client types and is able to communicate knowledge, experience, skills and attitude effectively and is at ease with different client-types. In short, a personal trainer must have and continue to cultivate excellent people-skills. It is important for personal trainers to muster soft skills like excellent listening and questioning, and acquire emotional quotient (people-skills and empathy) and adversity quotient (capability to bounce back after set-backs).

1.2.4 *A teacher and mentor*

A teacher should be a facilitator of learning and he/she must be knowledgeable in the exercise sciences- exercise physiology, sport medicine and injury prevention, basic and exercise nutrition, physical education, exercise and training technique and regimens, anatomy and sport biomechanics- as they are better informed about how exercise can affect the body. To teach is to touch someone's life forever. So teach to make a positive difference. The personal trainer is a mentor as they help clients approach their wellness goals in a safe, more efficient and streamlined manner. A main task of personal trainers is to help clients achieve a more positive state of physical change. The personal trainer does this by educating, empowering and fostering independence in their clients.

1.2.5 *Looks and acts professionally*

Personal trainers must dress and conduct themselves professionally at all times and steer clear of controversial dealings or communication with clients. They must be loyal but must never allow the mentor-client relationship to develop beyond that. They must be effective communicators and be able to market their services effectively but must be careful not to sell exercise products or nutritional supplements. They must practise what they preach- they do not smoke or drink excessively, they look good, are fit and healthy- in mind, body and action.

1.2.6 *Works with clients to set realistic wellness goals*

What is realistic is dependent on (i) the genetic potential of the client, (ii) the current state of wellness of the client, (iii) the time, motivation and commitment that the client can afford, and (iv) the interaction effects of (i), (ii) and (iii). A qualified personal trainer can develop a safe and effective exercise and nutrition programmes that can produce sustainable results. An important starting point is for the personal trainer to forge an agreement on what is achievable during the period of engagement. A good personal trainer is one who is great motivator and understands the process and stages of change and is able to guide and provide support or scaffolding to clients through the stages of change.

1.2.7 *Tactful but remains truthful*

Honesty and truthfulness are always a good policy. Part of being a personal trainer is to educate clients about dishonest products and gimmicks and unhealthy practices like weight-loss pills and body-building drugs, whilst remaining tactful to clients. Take a scientific and evidence-based stance to new exercise and nutritional products or practices.

1.2.8 *Pays attention to details of programming and quality of instruction*

The 'devil and angel' of quality personal training lie in the details, hence paying careful attention and being meticulous and organised can mean success or failure, between excellence and mediocrity, between stagnation and progress as a personal trainer. Programming can have many components: cardiovascular endurance, weight control, strength training, flexibility and sports specific training (coordination, speed, skill acquisition). A good personal trainer adjusts the combinations according the clients' life activities, goals and needs. Under promise and over deliver on the clients' needs. A good personal trainer is attentive and observant when instructing clients and is on a lookout for potential dangers in the gym or exercise area. A good personal trainer is conversant and apt with programme evaluation so as to fine-tune and make adjustments to suit the client's progress.

1.2.9 *Clients have more control over their lives and actions than you*

Personal trainers are teachers and mentors but they cannot make physical changes on behalf of their clients. They must educate their clients to take personal responsibility in daily effort (PRIDE) for making a physical change for the better, with the help of the personal trainer. Personal trainers help make it happen only when the client decides to make it happen.

1.2.10 *Runs a business like one*

Treat personal training like your own business. That means maintaining good paperwork, phone, communication and marketing procedures and website updated, filing away consent and indemnity forms, and client records, and keeping insurance and tax records current.

1.3   Personal Training Start-Up 101

1.3.1   *Is personal training my cup of tea?*

Honestly answer the following questions:

- ❖ Are you a people person?
- ❖ Are you a leader or a follower?
- ❖ Are you comfortable speaking in front of people?
- ❖ Are you an AM or PM person?
- ❖ Do you have lots of initiative?

If you answered 'yes' to all or many of the questions, then you have the right attributes or are willing to develop them. You must definitely be a people-person if you wish to be a successful personal trainer. Personal trainers must enjoy being leaders and most training takes place before or after work, and over the weekends too and so a great deal of sacrifice is in order. Personal trainers must be confident speaking in front of people and have ample initiative to get things going for the client.

1.3.2   *Get certified*

Experience is important but getting the appropriate certifications for personal training professionalises your service and helps you to stay current in the field. There are many certification bodies, but most are based overseas and on other contexts. The Singapore Sports Council, together with the National Institute of Education provides certification programmes for personal training. Getting a diploma or degree in exercise science or physical education together with a personal training certification will increase your confidence and help to bolster competence in knowledge and practice. Mainly clients are well-educated and would wish to work with trainers who are equivalent in intellect and with excellent people-skills.

1.3.3 *Make sure you have a current CPR certification*

CPR certification is a basic requirement as a personal trainer. Though you expect to work with healthy clients, exercise training may trigger off an emergency situation where you may need to perform CPR on your client. CPR can save lives on and off the job so do acquire a CPR certification and continue to keep it current and valid.

1.3.4 *Get the job by writing a good resume*

Like all jobs, writing a good resume and cover letter requires practice to get it right. Consider including the following headings:

- ❖ Goals - specify what motivates you as a personal trainer.
- ❖ Experience - number of clients, years of associated experience or practice.
- ❖ Certifications - list them clearly. Include the adult CPR certification.
- ❖ Training and Workshops - especially if they are specialist workshops on the latest training trends.
- ❖ Education - highest levels attained, special relevant professional qualifications.
- ❖ Achievements - were you employee of the month, a sports winner, completed a triathlon.
- ❖ Special Skills - know sign language, are bilingual, good with computers.

Get the order right and lead with your strengths first - what is different and outstanding about you compared to others. Let honesty drive your resume.

1.3.5 *Best part of being a personal trainer*

- ❖ Inspire clients.
- ❖ Transform bodies and minds.
- ❖ Keep own hours.

❖ Be your own boss.
❖ Change lives.
❖ Doing what you love.
❖ Earning more.

1.3.6 *Worst part of being a personal trainer*

❖ Clients missing appointments.
❖ Unmotivated clients with the same excuses.
❖ Irregular income.
❖ Pressure to sell gym memberships and meeting sales quotas.
❖ Clients wanting a magic pill not sound nutritional advice.
❖ Waking up early and getting home late.
❖ Missed weekends with family.
❖ Gossip partner, not trainer.
❖ Sexual harassment.

1.4 Start Your Own Business

You can get valuable information about starting your own business by using search engines and using key words. For example, to start your own business, you could first check out case examples of personal training websites (e.g. http://www.pt.com.sg/).

There are marketing agents out there that help you get ahead in terms of getting designing and marketing your website that gets you in the 10 ten sites whenever you someone sues the search engine on the internet to look for personal trainers.

1.5 Action Strategies

❖ Trawl newspaper, the internet and health magazines for the latest emerging health trends, exercise and training approaches, equipment and gadgets.
❖ Be an active practitioner by participating in exercise workshops or attending talks by recognised authorities in the field.

❖ Take an informed and scientific stance when it comes to controversial dietary and exercise practices.

❖ Practise active listening skills and positive body language by observing and mirroring the positive client posture and keeping in check negative body language and non-verbal cues.

❖ Keep all client information confidential and resist commenting on information that is heard and shared between clients.

❖ Practise and increase your vocabulary of words of motivation and practise marketing your services.

❖ Be a lifelong learner and take an interest in all things current. Spend at least an hour a week reading outside of your immediate area of expertise.

1.6   In the News

The Singapore Sports Council reported in the national press in April 2008 that the sports industry will be contributing two billion dollars to Singapore's GDP a year and will create another 20 000 jobs, up from 14 000 jobs in the sports and fitness industry by 2015. Personal training and coaching services will play a non-negligible part of the vibrant sports industry in Singapore now and in the years to come.

1.7   Summary and Key Points

A good personal trainer requires key competencies and personal dispositions that can be learned, practised and cultivated. It is really acquiring a strong knowledge in the area of fitness combined with excellent communication skills and a high dose of EQ. Three key commandments of personal training are noteworthy- (i) enhance the quality of life of the client, (ii) act like a caring and concerned friend training a valued colleague, and (iii) exercise knowledge, understanding and wisdom.

1.8   Recommended Readings and Website Resource

(1) Chia, M., Leong, L.L. and Quek, J.J. (2004). *Healthy, Well and Wise: Take PRIDE for a Life of Wellness.* National Institute of Education, Singapore. Order details: Office of Graduate Programmes and Professional Learning.

(2) Developed by a team of sport specialists from the National Institute of Education, SSSS is a scientific and holistic approach to understanding and practising the principles of science for conditioning for health and fitness. SSSS will help clients get the most out of their sporting pursuits, training, practice or competition. Harvesting success in sports is both an art and a science and paying heed to the contents of this website will equip clients with the knowledge to harnessing exercise talents safely and effectively: www.sportsuccess.nie.edu.sg

(3) Check out case examples of personal training websites in Singapore such as this website: www.pt.com.sg

(4) Find out more about personal training career information from: www.starting-a-personal-training-business.com/personal-trainer-career-info.html

Chapter 2

Code and Ethics of Personal Training

Professional ethics and code of conduct are important in personal training as they govern the way personal trainers behave and conduct themselves.

After completing this chapter, you will be able to:

❖ Know the general code of conduct and ethics for personal training.

❖ Practise the basic code of conduct and ethics for personal training.

❖ Understand that there are professional, regional and cultural differences in ethics of personal training.

2.1 Introduction

Personal trainers are entrusted with guiding and mentoring clients to better and improved physical health and are therefore expected to uphold the highest standards of integrity and professional behaviour, when dealing with clients or running a personal training business.

Physicians, lawyers, teachers and nurses or well-regarded professions have their own professional code of ethics or conduct where breaches of the code may result in loss of the license to practice as a professional, and in some cases, criminal prosecution.

A professional code of ethics for personal trainers, when subscribed and practised by all, will enhance the image of personal trainers and importantly, safeguard the best interests of clients. Remember that guarding your clients' best interest is good for your business.

The code may be updated as and when the need arises owing to circumstances of personal training practices within the profession, for example, in response to a greater need for legal client protection.

The general code of ethics and conduct for personal training may be categorised as (i) Safeguarding client interest (ii) Keeping professional boundaries (iii) Staying current in professional knowledge (iv) Letting truth and fairness guide all professional decisions, (v) Respecting all clients and fellow professional personal trainers and (vi) Maintaining a professional image.

2.2 Code and Practice

2.2.1 *Code 1: Safeguard the best interest of your client*

- ❖ The primary responsibility of the personal trainer is to protect and safeguard the client's safety, health and well-being. Never compromise this with your own self-gain, personal interest or monetary gain.
- ❖ Recommend products or services only if it benefits the client, not because it will boost your income or position.
- ❖ Disclose to your client any potential benefit that you will gain from selling products or services to your client.
- ❖ Base the number of training sessions required on your clients' needs and not your financial requirements.

2.2.2 *Code 2: Keep professional boundaries*

- ❖ Do not exploit any professional relationship with a client, supervisor, employee or colleague- sexually or economically.
- ❖ Always respect your client's right to privacy. A client's results, conversations, behaviour, secrets and where possible, even identity should be kept confidential.
- ❖ Focus on the professional trainer-client relationship and not the client's personal life, except when appropriate (e.g. when client is sharing his/her exercise or health history).

❖ Avoid any unnecessary physical contact or sexually-based banter with the client.

❖ When you are unable to maintain a professional relationship either because of your own limitations or that of the client, kindly refer him/her to another better equipped personal trainer or medical professional as appropriate.

2.2.3 Code 3: Stay current in professional knowledge

❖ Continually strive to stay abreast of all new developments in personal training practice and service delivery so as to provide scientific and evidence-based information to clients.

❖ Refer clients to other health care professionals, such as another personal trainer, doctor or mental health specialist, if a service required falls outside of your expertise. Recognise your limitations in expertise and only provide services that you are qualified to deliver.

❖ Adhere to guidelines and standards provided by professionals in the fields of medicine, health and fitness for health screening, fitness assessment, exercise progression and technique.

2.2.4 Code 4: Let truth and fairness guide all professional decisions

❖ Represent your credentials and qualifications accurately.

❖ When advertising your services, be guided by helping your client make informed decisions, judgments, opinions and choices.

❖ Make your contract language clear and simple.

❖ Be consistent in your fees for your services.

❖ Never solicit business from another trainer's client. When interacting with other trainer's clients, be open and honest so that clients cannot interpret the interaction as a solicitation of business.

❖ If you work for a fitness facility that recruits and assigns clients to you, respect that the clients belong to the business and not to you.

2.2.5 *Code 5: Respect clients and fellow professionals*

❖ Act professionally and respectfully towards all clients, colleagues and fellow fitness professionals so that the highest standards of service are secured for your clients.

❖ Do not discriminate based on race, nationality, religion, occupation, sex or educational background.

❖ When disagreements occur, focus on the behaviour and factual evidence not on 'heresay', placement of blame or on judgmental statements.

❖ Provide fitness and health-related information factually and accurately so that clients can make an informed decision or choice.

❖ Base fitness or product information on scientific evidence and not on testimonies of consumers or personal testimony.

2.2.6 *Code 6: Keep and uphold a professional image in dress and behaviour*

❖ Dress and behave appropriately so that clients are comfortable.

❖ Practise healthy habits- do not smoke or drink excessively on and off work.

❖ Keep fit and practise appropriate eating habits.

2.3 Action Strategies

❖ Subscribe to sport science journals or newsletters that are available free on-line.

❖ Keep abreast by reading the health and lifestyle sections of the national newspaper and supplements (e.g. Mind Your Body).

❖ Read at least one article per week in any area that is associated with medicine, sports science or healthcare. Make a record of them for future reference.

❖ Hold off commenting or gossiping on and off work about clients, colleagues or employers.

❖ Dress smart and always act appropriately. Remember that you are your best advertisement.

2.4 Summary and Key Points

Personal trainers should dress and behave professionally, use truth to guide all professional and relational decisions, seek to keep abreast of scientific and health developments, adhere to scientific principles of training and knowledge, guard against false practices, gossip or loose talk that compromises the confidentiality of clients, colleagues or employers and strive to act in the best interest of clients.

2.5 Recommended Readings and Website Resource

(1) Health supplements of newspapers, on-line health and fitness journals.

(2) Chia, M., Leong, L.L. and Quek, J.J. (2004). *Healthy, Well and Wise: Take PRIDE for a Life of Wellness.* National Institute of Education, Singapore. Order details: Office of Graduate Programmes and Professional Learning.

(3) Developed by a team of sport specialists from the National Institute of Education, SSSS is a scientific and holistic approach to understanding and practising the principles of science for conditioning for health and fitness. SSSS will help clients get the most out of their sporting pursuits, training, practice or competition. Harvesting success in sports is both an art and a science and paying heed to the contents of this website will equip clients with the knowledge to harnessing exercise talents safely and effectively: www.sportsuccess.nie.edu.sg

Chapter 3

The First Client Meeting — Keeping It Real

The best start is a start well-started. After completing this chapter, you will be able to:

- ❖ Prepare for a best start in personal training.
- ❖ Making sure the client is well-informed and empowered about his/her health status.
- ❖ Always be prepared- rehearse that first client meeting.

3.1   The Right Start

3.1.1   *Cardio Pulmonary Resuscitation (CPR) certification*

This is the most basic certification and even though most personal trainers work with healthy clients, it may sometimes be necessary to perform CPR on the client. Having a current CPR certification will also ensure that legal liability is kept to a minimal and it is also good for enhancing professional image of trainers and fostering client confidence in personal trainers.

3.1.2   *Emergency action plan*

If working in a fitness facility, the emergency action plan should be practised and become familiar to all personal trainers. Emergency phone numbers should always be visible and available and the nearest routes to hospitals should be checked out when the training is off-site.

3.1.3 *Health screening for risk factors*

This health screen should be provided by a medical physician which includes the following- major risk factor identification, personal medical history, current medication (if any), physician-determined contraindications for exercise, cardiovascular risk profile, and chronic illness or joint problems. Once clearance to exercise and partake in physical training is obtained and when it is assessed that personal training will not pose a risk of harm to the client, the trainer can start to explain the business policies and discuss the mutual expectations of personal training to the client.

3.1.4 *Physical activity readiness*

Clients should complete a standard Physical Activity Readiness Questionnaire (PAR-Q). The form informs the client and the personal trainer if additional medical clearance or advice is required before embarking on any supervised or unsupervised fitness programme.

3.1.5 *Personal particulars*

These should include name, age, sex, body mass, stature and body mass index, phone contact and address of the client. It should also include the contact of a nominated person in case of an emergency that involves the client.

3.1.6 *Informed consent and professional waiver*

Informed consent by the client means that the personal trainer has discussed with the client, the possibility of injury or even death when participating in the fitness programme. An Indemnity Form indemnifies the personal trainer from legal liability should any harm befall the client when participating in the fitness programme.

3.1.7 *Payment policies*

These could include:

- ❖ Monthly or per session or per hour fees.
- ❖ Contract-period based.
- ❖ Special packages for out-site or home visits.
- ❖ Policies for payment in advance, loss or missed session or cancellation.

3.1.8 *Mutual expectations*

These should be explicitly spelt out and acknowledged by the client and the personal trainer with a signed agreement. Details may include but is not limited to:

- ❖ What the client can expect from the personal trainer.
- ❖ What the personal trainer expects from the client.
- ❖ Termination or refund policies.
- ❖ Vacation plans (interruptions), bonuses or tardiness (late-coming) policies.

3.1.9 *Scheduling*

Consider including information about:

- ❖ Are training sessions in the morning, afternoon or evening?
- ❖ Are training sessions fixed at stipulated times or are they flexible and variable?
- ❖ What is the frequency and regularity of training? Twice a week? Every other day?
- ❖ Does training include travelling time and therefore additional transport fees?
- ❖ What is the duration of a typical training session? 45 minutes or 90 minutes?

3.2   Determining Client Goals and Limitations

Pay careful information to:

- ❖ Client goal categories- developing or improving cardiovascular, strength, weight maintenance, etc).
- ❖ Goal attainment time frames- short, medium and longer-term.
- ❖ Client personal information- name, age sex, height, weight, circumference- waist, hip, arms, legs, trunk, occupation, sleeping habits, water and food intake.

Other programming details could include:

- ❖ Special considerations or preference for fitness.
- ❖ Previous exercise or fitness history.
- ❖ Contraindications for exercise.

3.3   Formalising Forms

There are no hard and fast rules about how the forms should be constructed and put together but some thought should go toward not getting the client to fill in too many forms. Nonetheless, it is important to have proper documentary proof of client records, health and fitness status, goal agreements and business agreement and transactional records.

Some forms for consideration include:

- ❖ Policy and client agreement.
- ❖ Physical activity readiness questionnaire.
- ❖ Medical questionnaire.
- ❖ Waiver of liability.
- ❖ Exercise or workout history.
- ❖ Activity log.
- ❖ Client performance tracking.

Always be ready with a brochure, business card, resume and copies of your certifications including CPR.

3.4 Action Strategies

Always be punctual, smile a lot, smell nice and dress professionally. Be attentive to your client. Providing a glass of water and some fresh mints to the client will flavour the session.

3.5 Summary and Key Points

Getting organised at the start and keeping good records at the back end will help reduce the likelihood of client misunderstanding or conflict at the front end. This also instils confidence in the client and projects a positive image of personal trainers.

Chapter 4

Effective Fitness Programme Design

The constituents of effective fitness programme design include- record of client information, progressive resistance training, flexibility training, cardiovascular training, and balanced nutrition.

After completing this chapter, you will be able to:

- ❖ Know the constituents and benefits of a holistic fitness programme.
- ❖ Understand the general principles of training.
- ❖ Be aware of overtraining.
- ❖ Incorporate cross-training.
- ❖ Have knowledge of basic sports science.
- ❖ Understand special considerations when training indoors and outdoors.

4.1 Introduction

The art of programme design encapsulates meeting clients' needs- this involves knowing the medical, family and fitness history of the client through active listening, understanding and educating and addressing clients' needs and limitations. Effective fitness design necessitates having a comprehensive knowledge of the energy systems, human movement, biomechanics and motor control, sport psychology and the principles of fitness training- i.e. knowledge of basic exercise science concepts.

4.2 Holistic Physical Fitness

Constituents of holistic health components of physical fitness are listed below.

4.2.1 *Body composition*

Proportions of fat, muscle, bone and body fluids in the body. Apart from body fluid variation (up to 1 kg), fat and muscle mass are the most amenable to change with any sound exercise programme. Surrogate measurements of body composition include, body mass index, waist-to-hip ratio, and sum of skinfolds of body sites.

Goals for body composition should be to maintain or increase muscle mass or to reduce body fat and also to increase or preserve bone mass. A high percentage of body fat increases the risk of heart-disease and certain cancer forms.

4.2.2 *Muscular strength and endurance*

This is the maximum amount of force that a muscle (s) can generate or the number of times a muscle (s) can contract generate force. Goals for muscle endurance and muscle strength should focus on muscle balance and improving on areas of weakness.

4.2.3 *Cardiovascular endurance*

This is the capability to perform sustained exercise that involves large muscle groups (upper and lower limbs, torso) over extended periods of time (> 20 minutes at a stretch). Goals for cardiovascular fitness can include improving cardiovascular health (exercise duration > 20 minutes) or cardiovascular fitness (exercise duration > 30 minutes).

4.2.4 *Joint flexibility*

This is the range of motion of major joints. Goals for joint flexibility can include improving the flexibility of tight muscles and daily stretching to improve blood circulation and to enhance relaxation of the major muscle groups.

4.2.5 *Integrating fitness with nutritional programming*

A holistic fitness and exercise development plan is best integrated with a sound nutritional programme to accrue optimal benefits to the client. A balanced and well-nourished diet will ensure a proper recovery following training and in the longer term provide for an appropriate weight maintenance.

4.3 Muscle Strength and Endurance Conditioning

Personal trainers should encourage clients to have a balanced whole body muscle endurance and strength. Involve multi-muscle group exercises that are functional in daily life in each workout so that there is improved overall conditioning. Work both the agonist and the antagonist (e.g. chest and back). Work muscles that support the core- that means performing functional exercises like push-ups and squats in good form. Benefits of resistance training include increased muscle mass, increased resting metabolism, better muscle tone and greater functional strength for work and leisure.

4.4 Body Composition Monitoring

Aim for a gradual change in body composition, and increase muscle mass and reduce fat mass, if the client's body composition warrants it. Safe weight loss or safe weight gain should not be at a rate of more than 0.5 kg per week. Rapid weight loss is usually water loss as real changes in body composition takes weeks and months.

Gradual weight loss or gain will allow the body to get accustomed to the new exercise and dietary regimens being adopted and are most sustainable over the longer term. The benefits of an acceptable BMI are reduced risks of cardiovascular disease, stroke, hypertension and some cancer forms.

Table 4.1. The International Task Force For Obesity (IOTF) classification for Asians and World Health Organisation (WHO) classification for obesity for Europids are summarised.

IOTF classification of BMI categories for Asians	
BMI (kg/m^2)	Classification
Less than 18.5	Underweight
18.5-22.9	Normal
23.0-24.9	At risk of obesity
25.0-29.9	Obese I
Greater than 30.0	Obese II
WHO classification of BMI categories for Europids	
Less than 18.5	Underweight
18.5-24.9	Normal
25.0-29.9	Pre-obese
30.0-34.9	Obese I
35.0-39.9	Obese II
Greater than 40.0	Obese III

4.5 Cardiovascular Conditioning

Personal trainers should plan for aerobic type exercise such as brisk-walking, jogging, swimming or cycling 3-5 days per week for between 20-60 minutes per session at between 60-90% of maximum heart rate.

Beginners should start at the lower end of the prescription (2-3 days per week, 20 minutes per session, and exercising at 60% of max HR) and gradually build this up.

The formula below, while useful and simple to compute, does not take into consideration the cardiovascular fitness level of clients.

❖ Maximum heart rate (Max HR) is given by 220-Age (in years)
❖ Appropriate training intensity is 0.6 (220-Age) to 0.9 (220-Age)

A more sensitive training intensity for aerobic conditioning is using the Karvonen Formula. The desired training percentage for this formula is 50-85%

❖ Max HR-Rest HR X (0.5-0.85) + Rest HR

Use the talk test to estimate exercise intensity. A client should be able to hold a short conversation without being too breathless when exercising. If talking becomes increasingly difficulty, the exercise intensity is probably too hard. Personal trainers should teach beginners this useful tip as it 'educates' and empowers the client to take responsibility for listening to his/her body whilst exercising.

4.5.1 *Types of cardiovascular conditioning*

❖ *Fixed steady state exercise intensity* - Running or swimming at fixed relative exercise intensity for 20 minutes or more. Gradually progress to 30-60 minutes.

❖ *Interval training* - High intensity running for 10-15 minutes, interspersed with 10-15 minutes of low intensity walking or rest, repeated several times in the training session.

❖ *Speed play or Fartlek* - Speed of running is varied at different stages or durations depending on how the client feels on the day. Slope or gradient of running can be used to vary the pace.

4.5.2 *Benefits of aerobic conditioning*

These include improved mood, stress relief, improved aerobic fitness, improved blood profile, healthy blood pressure management, better quality sleep, a higher energy turnover, and weight loss or weight maintenance.

4.6 Joint Flexibility Conditioning

Stretching is often the most neglected segment of personal training. Conditioning for flexibility is important as it allows for a whole range of motion of the muscles and joints, keeps muscles pliable and prevents injury. Stretching also improves blood circulation and promotes muscle relaxation. Stretching can be done at anytime and anywhere and also follows the general principles of training like overload and progression. Stretch specific muscle groups that had been exercised. Stretching is best done following warm up and during cool down after exercise.

More details are presented in Chapter 5 Designing the Flexibility Programme. General tips for stretching include the following:

- ❖ Warm up muscles before stretching.
- ❖ Select a safe and comfortable place to stretch.
- ❖ Adopt the proper posture for each specific muscle stretch.
- ❖ Never stretch beyond mild tension.
- ❖ Gradually ease into a stretch and not force a stretch.
- ❖ Hold a stretch for at least 10 seconds, work towards 20-60 seconds.
- ❖ Breathe normally while stretching.

4.7 General Principles of Training

There are general principles of training that interact with the client's genetic make-up, fitness training history, motivation and commitment for training and the peculiarities of training programmes for strength, endurance, cardiovascular and flexibility to produce very varied outcomes among different clients. It is the personal trainer's job to help clients to navigate the training regimen to produce the most optimal fitness results.

Every personal trainer must be conversant with the following principles of training:

4.7.1 *Overload*

There must be exposure over a period of time in terms of an appropriate amount of exercise effort (strength, endurance, flexibility) if there is to be any gain in fitness. Safe overload exposures are within 10-30% of what is accustomed by the client on a daily basis.

4.7.2 *Progression*

For improvements in fitness, there must be progressions in overload and in the complexity of the exercise. These progressions should be advanced only when the client is accustomed to the overload. This usually takes about 4 to 6 weeks.

4.7.3 *Specificity*

Fitness gains are specific to the overload, even though there may be cross-training effects. For example, a circuit training programme that is designed for developing muscular fitness for the lower limbs will not result in improvements in muscular fitness for the upper limbs but may have some cardiovascular improvements because the time spent between stations is limited.

4.7.4 *Continuity*

For sustainability of fitness, there must be regularity of training. This will also habituate clients to the routine such that it comes part of the client's schedule of life.

4.7.5 *Rest, recovery and adaptation*

Rest and recovery between exercise bouts are essential for a period of physiological adjustment and adaptation so that the bodily systems become better and fitter in handling future exercise demands. Rest and recovery are also essential for the body to get rid of exercise metabolites and for the body to replenish muscle nutrients and for the body to repair bodily wear and tear.

4.7.6 *Individualisation*

Up to 50% of the physical fitness differences between people are explained by genetics. No two people will respond identically to the same exercise programme. Hence it is important to personalise and individualise the exercise programme to suit each client. A one-size-fits-all exercise programme should not be used for all clients.

4.7.7 *Reversibility or reversion*

This principle explains that training or overload exposure must be continued for fitness gains to be maintained. The removal of the overload stimulus of more than 48 hours means that fitness will start to decay to the initial levels of fitness that the body is accustomed to. Use it or lose it is operational in the principle of reversibility or reversion.

4.7.8 *Diminishing returns*

Early enthusiasm in training can mean that a client abuses the rest and recovery principle and over-trains, over-reaches or over-stretches, thereby resulting in less or reduced gains for the same exercise effort. Signs of over-training include sleeplessness, an increase in resting heart rate of more than 10 beats per minute, listlessness and lethargy, increased susceptibility to coughs and colds, and weight loss.

4.7.9 *Stagnation and plateauing*

Rates of improvements in fitness are dependent on the initial level of fitness at the beginning of the programme. Rates of improvements are usually greater for a client whose entry level of fitness is low compared to one whose fitness level is higher. Improvements in fitness may also plateau or stagnate if the overload is inadequate or when the programme becomes 'stale'. Reassessing training goals or introducing a variety of training may be appropriate when there is stagnation.

4.7.10 *Variety, mixed or cross-training*

The involvement of different routines such exposure to different forms of weight resistance training (free, machines, body weight), flexibility exercises (static, PNF), and cardiovascular training (interval, continuous,

Fartlek) will provide for variety and motivation for the client. Cross-training (mixed training) is usually introduced to provide for balance and variety and is usually introduced in the 'off-season' for competitive athletes.

4.7.11 *Periodisation*

Periodising the training programme provides for the opportunity for 'peaking' or optimizing fitness returns when it matters most such as during competition.

4.8 Overtraining

When clients are enthusiastic and have experienced some measure of success in terms of improvements in fitness, personal trainers must be mindful of the dangers of overtraining. The following are some of the signs of overtraining:

- ❖ Prolonged muscle soreness.
- ❖ Irritability.
- ❖ Depressed immune system hence increased susceptibility to colds and the common flu.
- ❖ A lack of motivation to exercise or taking a long time to complete a training routine.
- ❖ Fatigue and general malaise.
- ❖ Depression.
- ❖ An increase of a resting heart rate of more than 10 beats per minute.

If a client is over-stretched or over-reached, take a break from the training routine, encourage the client to have an active rest and to eat a high carbohydrate diet. Re-evaluate the training programme thereafter.

Personal trainers should constantly communicate with clients and be on the look-out for signs and symptoms of over-reaching. This communicates to the client that the trainer is sensitive and responsive to the needs of the client. Remember the key criteria for quality service delivery are reliability, responsiveness, reassurance, tangible outcomes and empathy.

4.9 Incorporate Variety, Mixed or Cross-Training

It is said that variety is the spice of life and this is no different when it comes to conditioning for fitness. By varying the mode (or type) of training, intensity of training, venue of training and mixing different forms of training, the client is provided with variety and balance. This helps keep boredom from setting into the exercise routine and helps with exercise adherence. Sportsmen often use cross-training, especially during the off-season to infuse freshness into training.

Table 4.2. A sample cross-training programme for a beginner.

Day	Activity	Duration
Monday	❖ Slow jogging on the treadmill at 6-8 km/hr ❖ Upper body muscle group stretching ❖ Resistance training for the upper body	❖ 20 mins ❖ 15 mins ❖ 30 mins
Wednesday	❖ Steady pace jogging ❖ Lower body muscle group stretching ❖ Resistance training for the lower body	❖ 30 mins ❖ 15 mins ❖ 30 mins
Friday	❖ Pilates or Yoga or core muscle training	❖ 60 mins

4.10 Understanding Basic Sports Science

This segment provides a revision and an overview of the major concepts in sports science that are useful to know and revise for use in personal training.

4.10.1 *Energy systems*

The energy needs of all exercise are met by the interplay of the three energy systems. These are the Phosphagen Energy System, the Lactic Acid Energy System and the Oxygen Energy System.

The Phosphagen Energy System is the main source of energy provision when the exercise is explosive and short in duration (usually within 30s). The Lactic Acid Energy System provides most of the energy when the exercise task is of a moderate-to-high intensity and last for less than 2 minutes, while the Oxygen Energy System provides energy for exercise that is of a low to moderate intensity and lasts for more than 2 minutes, up to several hours.

The main energy source of the Phosphagen Energy System is stored Adenosine Triphosphate and Creatine Phosphate (ATP-CP) in the muscles.

The main energy source for the Lactic Acid Energy System is muscle glycogen, a stored form of carbohydrate. The main energy source of the Oxygen Energy System is free fatty acids.

In the context of personal training, training for cardiovascular fitness focuses the training of the oxygen-delivery and aerobic metabolism mechanisms of the Oxygen Energy System. Weight training for muscle endurance or strength draws mainly from, and therefore trains the ATP-CP and Lactic Acid Energy Systems.

4.10.2 *Factors that affect contribution of the energy systems*

4.10.2.1 *Genetics*

All human beings are unique. Some of us may be more gifted in powerful activities (well-developed ATP-CP & Lactic Acid energy systems) while others may be more gifted in endurance type activities (well-developed oxygen system).

Most world class sportsmen are naturally gifted in one way or another. However most of us are reasonably balanced in terms of the genetics of the energy system-that is we can perform both power (fast) and endurance (slow) type activities reasonable well, but not exceeding well. Some research suggests that genetics contribute about 50-90% of our exercise capabilities.

4.10.2.2 *Sex*

Some data show that girls and women are most suited to aerobic-type activities, while boys and men perform better in power-type activities. However, some of these obvious sex differences are reduced when body size, especially muscle mass is taken into account. Male adults have 15-25% more muscle mass than female adults.

4.10.2.3 *Age, development and maturity*

The three energy system components are not fully developed until late adulthood. For instance performance data suggest that the oxygen system and lactic acid systems reach their maximal potential between 25 and 35 years of age. Children before puberty are less capable of performing high intensity exercise due to a less developed lactic acid system and they do not tolerate a high level of lactic acid in the blood as well as adults.

4.10.2.4 *Exercise intensity*

When the exercise intensity is low, the energy needs of the body can be met by mainly by the oxygen system. However as the exercise intensity increases, there will be increased contribution to the energy supply from the lactic acid system and when the intensity increases to maximal effort, there will also be energy contribution from the ATP-CP system. During 'start and go' activities, there is a great deal of overlap in energy supply from both aerobic and anaerobic sources.

4.10.2.5 *Exercise duration*

Less than 30s-the effort is all out- the energy is provided mainly by the ATP-CP system (anaerobic). Between 30s and 3 minutes-the exercise effort is intense- the energy is provided mainly by the lactic acid system. Greater than 3 minutes-the exercise effort is low to moderate- the energy is provided mainly by the oxygen system.

4.10.2.6 *Specific training*

Appropriate and specific training of the energy systems will fine-tune and enhance the capability of the system to provide energy when it is required.

4.10.2.7 *Fitness levels*

A person with a high level of anaerobic fitness will be able to accomplish tasks which demand high power while someone with a high level of aerobic fitness will be able to accomplish tasks which require high exercise endurance.

A person with a balanced fitness development will be able to accomplish a higher level of exercise effort all round and also recover swiftly from the exercise efforts.

4.10.2.8 *Fatigue or sleep deprivation*

The energy system is negatively affected because of fatigue or a lack of sleep. This means that adequate recovery time between training sessions is important for the energy system to adjust and adapt to the training.

4.10.2.9 *Diet and nutrition*

A balanced diet is essentially for the energy system to function optimally. This can be accomplished by paying careful attention to what you eat or drink before, during and after exercise.

4.10.2.10 *Illness and disease*

Illness and disease usually negatively affect energy supply from all the components of the energy system. Therefore one should not exercise when ill or unwell. Also progress gradually again when training after a period of illness.

Get a doctor's clearance to exercise when you are living with a disease. This is important as you will be advised specially about what you can do and what you should avoid because of the disease.

4.10.2.11 *Environment*

When exercising in the heat, cold or at altitude (i.e. greater than 1500m), there is usually an increase in energy supply from the lactic acid system until acclimatization to the heat, cold or altitude occurs. This is usually accomplished in days or weeks with appropriate exercise exposure to the environment.

4.10.3 *Diet and nutrition*

The best diet for all situations for an active and healthy client is a balanced diet- that means paying attention to the quality and quantity of the daily diet- food and drink.

It is good advice to eat a wide variety of foods from all food groups-rice and alternatives (carbohydrate- 6-7 servings daily), meat and alternatives (protein and fat, minerals- 2 servings daily), fruit and vegetable (vitamins, minerals and fibre- 2 servings each daily) and dairy products and alternatives (minerals- 2 servings daily).

It is important to match and moderate eating habits to energy output (daily physical activity, including exercise and physical recreation), with less physically active people eating less.

Water is also an important part of a balanced diet and most should drink about 2 litres of water daily or more to keep the colour of the urine, a very pale yellow or colourless throughout the day.

4.10.4 *Stability and lever arm*

Keeping the centre of mass of the client, within the base of support or extending the base of support, provides greater stability than standing tall (raising the centre of mass) or allowing the centre of mass to fall out of the base of support. Hence, seated exercise provides greater stability than standing exercise, or standing with feet a stride increases the base of support compared to standing with feet together when performing dumbbell exercises.

Keeping the arms close centre of mass (shorter lever arm) when lifting weights makes the exercise safer and easier than raising the arms away from the centre of mass, rotation or pivot point, whilst lifting the weight. Hence when lifting weights, it is safely to keep the weight close to the body and using multi-muscle groups (e.g. muscles in the upper and lower limbs).

4.10.5 *Stages of learning*

The stages of learning include beginner (novice), intermediate (in-between) and autonomous (expert). The beginner stage is characterized by jerky and unsure movement patterns where many repetitions of the same exercise will help the novice reduce errors when performing the exercise. The personal trainer can help the novice by not over-explaining the exercise but instead allow for ample practice. The autonomous stage characterizes the experienced exercise performer where the personal trainer can help the client focus more on the quality or finer points of doing the exercise.

In terms of 'whole' versus 'part' learning in simple exercises, it is better to demonstrate the exercise as a whole rather than break it down into parts. More complex exercise routines may be broken down into simpler parts to facilitate skill acquisition. However, some clients may perform grasp better when the exercise is demonstrated as a whole while some others may do better when the exercise is broken down into parts.

In any case, visually demonstrating the exercise while verbalizing the explanation for the exercise is useful as it involves multiple senses of the client. Providing ample opportunity for the client to see the demonstration, listening to the explanation of the demonstration and mimicking the demonstration with expert feedback and encouragement are ingredients of good personal training.

4.10.6 *Stages of behaviour modification*

In terms of health behaviour change, 5 stages are proposed by Prochaska (1992).

❖ Stage 1: Pre-Contemplation- a lack of awareness with no intention to change behaviour. The personal trainer can provide up-to-date information to the client.

❖ Stage 2: Contemplation- consideration for change but without commitment to change. The personal trainer can help the client commit to a timeframe for action by mutually arranging appointments for exercise.

❖ Stage 3: Preparation- definite intention for deliberate action in the near future. The personal trainer can follow-up for appointments for exercise by reminding clients of the appointments.

❖ Stage 4: Action- behaviour modification in progress. The personal trainer can provide a meaningful experience by providing close and appropriate support during this stage.

❖ Stage 5: Maintenance- stabilization of the new behaviour and the avoidance of relapse. The personal trainer can continue to give encouragement and avoid staleness from creeping into the programme by providing for variety of training approaches.

Every client is different and may be at different stages of behaviour modification. Hence the personal trainer must be perceptive and provide the appropriate support and employ strategies that can help clients transit and move onto action and maintenance stages of behaviour modification.

4.11 Considerations When Training Outdoors

There are advantages and disadvantages of outdoors but the safety of the client is paramount. When training outdoors, pay attention to the following tips:

❖ Take along a first aid kit in case of emergencies.
❖ Be aware of any special medical conditions of the client- e.g. diabetic, asthmatic, on medication, etc.
❖ Make sure you know the location of the nearest hospital.

❖ If the client is asthmatic, ensure that he/she brings along an inhaler.

❖ Use sun-screen and make sure that the client is appropriately dressed for the outdoors, including proper shoes.

❖ Make sure the client has water or isotonic drinks.

❖ Have some energy bars available just in case.

❖ Take a fully charged mobile phone along.

❖ Inform park officers and the client's next-of-kin when going hiking.

4.12   Training in a Health Club

4.12.1   *Pros*

❖ Wider choice of equipment and programming is relatively easy.

❖ Clients prefer the social setting in the club.

❖ As a trainer, there is support from the administrators of the club.

❖ There is no additional travelling time for the trainer and he/she may have more clients.

4.12.2   *Cons*

❖ Clients are limited to members of the club.

❖ During peak hours the club, waiting time to use the equipment may be long.

❖ Some clients may be uncomfortable in a club setting.

❖ A gym setting does not mimic the activities of daily living and clients may not be motivated to exercise in an 'unnatural setting'.

❖ Trainers may have to pay a fee for using the club facility so the net income from personal training is less.

4.13 Training at Home

4.13.1 *Pros*

- ❖ There are no membership fees to be paid.
- ❖ Clients are more comfortable at home as there is more privacy.
- ❖ Client's time is maximized as they are at home.
- ❖ Clients become familiar with exercising with minimum equipment or can use modified equipment found in their home.
- ❖ Clients may feel more committed when a trainer visits them at home.

4.13.2 *Cons*

- ❖ Trainers must factor in travelling time in-between clients and may therefore have fewer clients.
- ❖ Clients may feel too comfortable at home as there may be other distractions like children, phone calls and pets.
- ❖ Trainers may need to invest in simple equipment like dumbbells, barbells, resistance bands and mats.
- ❖ Trainers may need a van or a car to transport the equipment so costs associated with transport must be factored into the personal training fee.

4.14 Action Strategies

- ❖ Practise and actualise balanced physical fitness by developing appropriate body composition, cardiovascular, muscular endurance and strength, and joint flexibility.
- ❖ Internalise and understand the basic principles of training and how they may apply to clients.
- ❖ Revise and internalise key concepts of exercise physiology, biomechanics, skill acquisition and exercise psychology.

4.15 In the News

Lifestyle physical activities are a good way to start on any exercise programme- check out the neighbourhood community clubs for a wide basket of mass and customised exercise and nutrition programmes. It is an excellent way to know the neighbourhood and make new friends to.

4.16 Summary and Key Points

Keep good and updated records of client information- risk assessment and medical clearance or exercise, PAR-Q, signed informed consent and client agreement on compliance and mutual expectations. A holistic fitness and exercise programme will include progressive resistance exercise, flexibility exercise, cardiovascular exercise and balanced nutrition. A firm grasp of the 11 principles of training and how they apply to various fitness programmes are a must. Basic sports science concepts useful in personal training include exercise physiology, exercise psychology, skill acquisition and exercise biomechanics.

4.17 Technology Updates

Step-counters and heart-rate monitors are useful devices for monitoring the volume and physical intensity of physical activity. These data can be used as an educational and motivational tool for the exercise programme. Bosu balance trainers are popular air-bladder devices that are useful for the development of core strength.

4.18 Recommended Readings and Website Resource

(1) Chia, M., Leong, L.L. and Quek, J.J. (2004). *Healthy, Well and Wise: Take PRIDE for a Life of Wellness.* National Institute of Education, Singapore. Order details: Office of Graduate Programmes and Professional Learning.

(2) Prochaska, J.O., et al. (1992). In search of how people change: applications to addictive behaviours, *American Psychology*, 47, pp. 1102–1114.

(3) Developed by a team of sport specialists from the National Institute of Education, SSSS is a scientific and holistic approach to understanding and practising the principles of science for conditioning for health and fitness. SSSS will help clients get the most out of their sporting pursuits, training, practice or competition. Harvesting success in sports is both an art and a science and paying heed to the contents of this website will equip clients with the knowledge to harnessing exercise talents safely and effectively: www.sportsuccess.nie.edu.sg

Part 2

Specific Programme Issues

Chapter 5

Designing the Flexibility Programme

An effective flexibility training programme is one that can address the client's areas of insufficient flexibility, muscle tightness, and/or postural misalignments. There are many benefits that can be gained from regular and deliberate flexibility or stretching workouts.

As a personal trainer, it is important to have a clear understanding on and sound knowledge of how to plan and formulate specific, safe and effective stretching exercises that can help the client. Flexibility training can definitely be a very enjoyable and relaxing part of the client's workout.

After completing this chapter, you will be able to:

- ❖ Understand health benefits of flexibility training.
- ❖ Understand anatomy of stretching.
- ❖ Understand basic principles for flexibility training.
- ❖ Demonstrate various stretching methods.
- ❖ Plan and instruct flexibility-based activities and safe effective stretching exercise.

5.1 Introduction

Having adequate flexibility is known to bring many positive benefits to individuals. Flexibility is often defined as the range of movement in a joint or in several joints, and is developed by stretching the soft tissues primarily around the joints. To the lay person, this would mean having the ability of a joint to move freely through its full normal range of motion.

In sports, there is an increasing awareness of the value of flexibility training and stretching to sports athletes as it can improve their overall sporting performance. However, the importance of flexibility in our daily lives and the value of flexibility training to physical fitness, functional health and overall wellness tend to be underestimated and poorly understood by the majority of the population.

This chapter unveils the health benefits that can be derived from flexibility training and stretching, discusses the anatomy of stretching, flexibility training methods, proper stretching techniques, and assessment approaches, as well as explores other safe and effective stretching activities suitable for most individuals.

5.2   Health Benefits of Improved Flexibility

If stretching is done occasionally, briefly and only concentrating on some muscle groups of the body, flexibility gains may not be optimised. For any person, adopting a regular stretching routine definitely can bring about many health benefits. Here is a list of the physiological and mental health benefits that can be gained:

5.2.1   *Better posture*

It is possible for the body to have adapted to habits of poor or incorrect postures over the years.   Poor exercise techniques can also lead to muscular imbalances and incorrect postural alignment. While flexibility training leads to improved flexibility, stretching exercises performed on a regular basis will also bring about increased muscular endurance and muscular strength. Clients will eventually experience improved muscular balance and find it easier to maintain proper posture and control their movements in sporting activities and daily chores.

5.2.2   *Better range of motion and functional flexibility*

With flexibility training, clients will develop the ability to exert greater force through a wider range of motion. A joint that is more mobile and moves more easily through a range of motion safely and effectively, whether in sporting activities or while performing daily chores, will exert less energy through greater mechanical efficiency.

5.2.3 *Injury prevention*

Flexibility is often seen as one of the best ways to prevent or avoid musculotendinous injuries. If muscles and tendons are inflexible, they are likely to be strained and injury to that part of the body will occur if movements are performed through range of motions beyond their limits. Research has shown that improved and sufficient flexibility and strength in the gluteus muscles, hamstrings, hip flexors and low back musculature reduce risk of lower back problems, and prevent or relieve joint pain that accompanies aging.

5.2.4 *Better circulation and relieve muscle stiffness*

Adequate warm-up and stretching exercises will bring about increased tissue temperature and improved blood circulation and nutrient delivery through the blood. For athletes, immediately after strenuous exercise or training, delayed onset muscle soreness (DOMS) can occur and may even be felt up to 48 hours after training. Slow, static stretching performed after exercise, and repeated stretching two or three times a day, can reduce or prevent delayed muscular soreness, alleviate the severity and duration of DOMS, and enhance recovery from exercise. An injury to a part of the body typically can cause tightening and stiffness of the muscles and tendons, and restricted movement around that joint. Gentle static stretching exercises, if done under proper supervision, can also aid faster recovery of the injury.

5.2.5 *Better relaxation and personal enjoyment*

Prolonged muscular tension tightens or shortens the muscles, making them less supple over time. Flexibility training or stretching exercises that form part of the cool down routine will help to prevent the muscles from tightening up and enhance muscular relaxation. Stretching when conducted in the proper environment also encourages personal enjoyment and mental relaxation, which can lead to a reduction of stress levels. Clients can learn to take their minds off work-related or other distracting issues while spending time stretching either by themselves or with others. Stretching together in a group may even create an opportunity for friendships and bonding in a relaxed atmosphere.

5.3 Anatomy of Stretching

The gain or loss of flexibility is highly specific to a joint. This also means that flexibility in one joint will not influence flexibility in other joints. Flexibility is influenced by various factors. Flexibility decreases with age, but is mainly attributed to a gradual loss of elasticity in the muscle. Nevertheless, for any beginner and even accompanying aging, it is still possible to develop some degree of flexibility in all joints with flexibility training.

Females tend to be more flexible than males, and this difference, which could exist throughout the adult life, is primarily due to anatomical variation in joint structures, for example, in the trunk and pelvic regions. As a result of growth and development from puberty, the decrease in flexibility for males is more related to greater increases in muscle size, muscle strength and stature.

The flexibility at a joint is limited by the structure of the joint itself and the physical properties of connective tissues, which could vary from joint to joint, and from person to person. The range of motion is primarily limited by one or more connective tissues of the joint including cartilages, ligaments, tendons and muscle fascia.

Ligaments and tendons are rich in protein collagen and therefore are more resistant to stretch (also can be described as having a high degree of elasticity). Muscle fascia which 'wraps' individual and groups of muscle fibers and whole muscles is less resistant to stretch. With adequate warm-up, tissue temperature increases and muscle fascia becomes warmed and stretchable.

As a result of flexibility training, improvement in the range of movement about a joint comes through two different types of connective tissue adaptation, namely elastic and plastic. In an elastic stretch, the tissue being stretched is able to return to its original length after the stretching force is removed. A plastic stretch, for example to the ligaments and tendons, will result in a 'permanent' and further elongation of the tissue being stretched.

Muscles have elastic properties, while ligaments and tendons have both elastic and plastic properties. If permanent increase in range of motion is desired, then flexibility training will target plastic deformation in the tissue. However, it is important that flexibility training workouts do not lengthen the ligaments surrounding the joint to a point that compromises joint stability.

In fact, in contact sports, athletes ought to be more careful not to overstretch their joints as they may become unstable and be easily injured. In cases where stretching forces are too great, a sprain (i.e. damage to ligamentous collagen fibers) or a muscle strain (i.e. damage to muscle fibers) can also happen.

Flexibility workouts that aim to maintain good posture and range of motion for daily living may be sufficient for most individuals. Very often, extreme ranges of motion and contorted stretch postures are high-risk for the majority of the population. It is therefore important that the personal trainer understands the client's flexibility needs and does not expose the client to unnecessary increased risk of injury. However, there is an extensive range of flexibility in the normal population.

For cases of hypomobility, flexibility exercises should commence with caution. Improvements to range of movements should not be rushed but rather gradually over an extended period of time. Hypomobility is mainly due to stiffness or unusual soft tissue tightness and often is more common among muscular individuals. It can also be due to abnormally large bony structures in the joint, tight joint capsules and bulky musculature.

Hypermobility, on the other hand, is characterized by excessive instability. If not careful during large extreme movements, it may lead to partial or complete dislocation easily. This is mainly due to loose joint capsules, ligaments, and also abnormally small bony structures in the joint. To decrease range of motion in hypermobile joints, the trainer can prescribe an intensive strength training programme which helps to tighten the surrounding muscles to give more support to the joint.

5.4 Basis Principles for Flexibility Training

5.4.1 *Teach proper techniques*

Stretching will not pose any risk to the body if stretching exercises are properly guided. Proper techniques must be taught to clients and must be practiced while the client performs the various stretching exercises. This will ensure that the flexibility training will be safe and effective to attain maximum benefits for the client. Stretching exercises that are not done in correct postural positions will put considerable pressure on the limbs and accompanying joints and may cause an injury.

5.4.2 *Stabilise the body before performing the stretch*

Stabilising the parts of the body before performing the stretch on the required muscles is necessary to prevent stretching the wrong muscles. For example, in stretching the quadriceps muscles, the knees are kept together or in line and the hip is either kept straight or pressed to the floor in the prone body posture to hold the pelvis in a neutral and stable position as a stretch is applied to the quadriceps muscle. More pictures of common stretches with their accompanied instructions on proper body or joint positioning are provided in the sections below.

5.4.3 *Make sure muscles are warm*

Stretching should be done after some activities that get the body to a light sweat (i.e. easy jogging, light cycling, etc). Flexibility training is most effective when muscles are warm. Nevertheless, it will be important to match the stretching exercises to the demands of the upcoming physical activity. If the upcoming activity is a leisurely jog, excessive stretching or bouncing movements will not be necessary. However, before any strenuous physical exercise or training, a minimum of 5 to 15 minutes stretching can be necessary to be incorporated as a part of the warm-up routine. Likewise, stretching can also be included as a part of the cool-down routine after exercise.

5.4.4 *Relax into the stretch*

Stretching should be done in a relaxed state. Ensure the area where stretching exercises are performed is quiet and away from distractions. Stretching on the floor with enough space or on an exercise mat can be reasonably comfortable. Clothing should be non-restrictive to allow stretching with ease. Finally, slow and even breathing while performing the stretch exercise keeps the body relaxed.

5.4.5 *Keep a comfortable amount of tension*

Usually, a comfortable amount of tension can be felt in the muscles being stretched. A proper and good stretch should not be painful. After holding stretch for at least 15 to 20 seconds, it is normal to feel a reduction in tension as the muscles being stretched lengthen. Often, the muscles may even feel warmer and looser after the stretch is being released.

5.4.6 *Keep client's safety, goals and needs as first priority*

When planning any flexibility training programme, always remember to keep the client's safety, goals and needs in first priority. Do not encourage clients to overstretch at any joints beyond the point of active control.

While it is possible to combine the various types of stretching into one programme, avoid ballistic or bouncy stretching exercises unless such exercises can meet client's specific needs, for example training for a particular sporting requirement.

Other than stretching as a part of the warm-up and cool-down routines, specifically performing stretching exercises for about 20 minutes or longer at least twice a week can also help the client to improve overall flexibility.

5.4.7 *Knowing where to stretch*

A common question asked by most clients has to do with which parts of
the body they should stretch. To an athlete, it will be necessary to stretch
the parts of the body subject to stress in a particular sport.

For a runner, this would mean spending more time stretching the hip,
thigh and leg muscles as compared to a swimmer, who will be making
sure the shoulder and back regions of the body are well stretched. Most
sporting movements will produce big bodily movements (i.e. netball,
tennis, biathlon, etc) that involve all body parts, thus will require
stretching to all parts of the body equally.

Generally, for most of the population not participating heavily in
sports, stretching to all parts of the body muscles will be necessary to
promote good posture and overall functional flexibility. It is possible that
tightness in one part of the body may put pressure on a nerve or other
anatomical structures, causing referred discomfort or tightness in a
muscle next to it.

A safe guideline to follow is to stretch the back and upper part of the
limbs first, then followed by the parts of the limbs furthest away from the
spine. For some clients, it may be more important to stretch more
frequently those muscles that are stiff – slow and gentle stretching can
relieve tension and stiffness.

Where there is muscle soreness and imbalance due to weight or
strength training, all the more stretching as part of warm up and cool
down in weight training routines cannot be skipped.

5.4.8 *Knowing when not to stretch*

If the client experiences any of these unusual symptoms (sharp pain,
numbness, tingling, swelling or burning sensation) while stretching, stop
the stretching exercise immediately. Other considerations include within
the first 24 to 72 hours of muscular or tendinous trauma, when joints or
muscles are infected or inflamed, stretching tissues or areas of the body
associated with an area of recent fracture, and if osteoporosis is present
or suspected.

5.4.9 *Seek professional advice if pain and discomfort persists*

There should not be a moment in flexibility training, or even in any other types of training programme, where the client is made to feel compelled to endure pain.

Make it a habit to ensure honest communication between the personal trainer and the client when it comes to subjective description of bodily discomfort experienced before, during and after exercise or training.

It is advisable to seek professional advice (i.e. sports medicine doctor, physiotherapist) should feelings of pain and numbness or swelling continue even after stretching. If stretches involving the spine produce pain, continuous stretching may make it worse. Where there is a suspicion a client is injured in any way some time back and has not sought professional advice, it is highly advisable to refer the client to see a doctor or physiotherapist for treatment.

5.5 Types of Flexibility Training

Flexibility exercises typically can be classified into three basic types:

- ❖ Static Stretching.
- ❖ Ballistic or Dynamic Stretching.
- ❖ Proprioceptive Neuromuscular Facilitation (PNF).

5.5.1 *Static stretching*

Static stretching is the most common method of stretching. It involves holding the stretched muscle in a still position for a period of time, usually between 15 and 30 seconds, with a constant stretching force being applied to it. Slow static stretching is safe and relatively effective in relaxing the muscles and the central nervous system when performed over a reasonable time, but should only be undertaken once the body is warm (i.e. after warm-up dynamic activity).

Static stretching will usually involve the following steps or pointers as shown in Table 5.1. Illustrations of common flexibility and stretching exercises can be found in Section 5.7 below.

Table 5.1. Useful steps or pointers for static stretching.

1	Holding a slow stretch for up to 30 seconds.
2	After holding the stretch for the initial 10 to 15 seconds, it is common to feel the stretch tension beginning to partially diminish. At which point, move into a deeper stretch and hold for another 10 to 15 seconds.
3	Each muscle should be stretched on each side of the body, alternate from left to right, at least two to three times. Do not stretch the same muscle twice or three times in a row. If a particular muscle or muscle group is seemingly tight, it may be better to stretch more than three times.

5.5.2 *Ballistic dynamic stretching*

Ballistic stretching involves putting a body segment through a range of motion by active contraction of a muscle group, and then over. The momentum of the movement is arrested by the antagonists at the end of the range of motion. In this way, the antagonists are stretched by the dynamic movements of the agonists. This type of stretching is also called "dynamic stretching". Watch out for the following guidelines when administering ballistic stretching in Table 5.2.

Table 5.2. Useful steps or pointers for ballistic dynamic stretching.

1	Make sure the muscles are thoroughly warm up before performing any ballistic stretches.
2	When starting off, keep the range of movement small and perform the action slowly and with control to get a feel of the motion before speeding up the action. Keep the average frequency to about one stretch per second.
3	Keep the movement in the desired direction and not drift out of alignment. Perform a stretch in series of 10 to 20, or more where necessary.

Stretching exercises used in sports in the past have been ballistic in nature and was only recently questioned on its suitability for to meet specific requirements as it could lead to injury and muscle soreness. If a sudden stretch is applied to the muscle, the muscle has a reflex action that causes it to contract. This then causes increased muscle tension, making it harder to stretch the connective tissue.

If ballistic stretching is necessary to meet a specific sporting requirement, especially true for sports that have a strong agility component and are ballistic in nature (i.e. jumping, sprinting, throwing, etc), and if it is done properly and with caution, it can be effective in increasing flexibility. However, for most of the population, this type of flexibility workouts may not be suitable and therefore need not be prescribed.

5.5.3 *Proprioceptive Neuromuscular Facilitation (PNF)*

PNF techniques are widely adopted in sports training. It has been suggested that PNF produces the best results in flexibility than the other types of flexibility training.

Table 5.3. Useful guidelines or tips for PNF stretching.

1	The body and muscles must be thoroughly warm up prior to applying PNF techniques.
2	The targeted muscle is initially placed in a lengthened position and hold for about 10 seconds, and then isometrically contracted against an immovable resistance from 6 to 10s. Resistance is usually provided by a partner (i.e. training partner or trainer).
3	The isometric contraction should not be performed explosively, but rather allow the contraction to gradually reach maximal effort within few seconds. While the muscle is contracted, the partner should not allow any joint movement at this stage.
4	After the isometric contraction phase, a brief period of relaxation followed, and after which a static stretch is taken into a new and further position and held for at least 10 to 30 seconds. An active or passive stretch can be applied at this static stage to complete the stretch.
5	If a passive force is applied after the brief period of relaxation, the partner needs to make sure the muscle is not overstretched. It is important to note here that the person being stretched must remain in control of the amount of stretch force being applied and feedback to the partner to avoid over stretching and injury. If the tension causes pain, stop immediately.
6	If an active stretch is first applied after the brief period of relaxation, there is a choice to complete the stretch here, or to complete the stretch with an addition passive stretch held at the subjective intensity of "comfortable discomfort" for another 10 to 60 seconds.
7	The process is repeated up to 3 to 4 times (in a series for each muscle), with each time achieving a further position.

Useful guidelines or tips to do PNF stretching properly are provided in Table 5.3. Whether PNF stretching is useful in personal training settings will depend on the specific goals and needs of the client. Since a partner is usually required when applying PNF techniques, the partner needs to be sufficiently trained to be able to handle the techniques safely with the client. Most of the time in a personal training setting, the person who assists the client with the PNF techniques is usually the personal trainer.

PNF involves a static stretch held in a lengthened position, followed by a strong isometric contraction held against an immovable resistance for few seconds, and followed by another stretch held in a further position. Due to certain reflex mechanisms in the muscle, a greater muscle relaxation can be achieved after a significant contraction of a muscle. The most common PNF technique is the "Contract-Relax-Contract" technique.

Below are two examples of common PNF stretches with a trainer or partner providing counter pressure. Notice how the body is being positioned with the body or parts of the body being stabilised before the stretch force on the required muscles is applied.

Example 1: Anterior deltoid and pectorals

❖ *Sequence A:* Using PNF technique, the trainer supports by placing the leg against the client's back, and pulls client's arms back to stretch pectorals at the first point of tension. Client resists the forward motion for 6-10 seconds.

❖ *Sequence B:* The pull on the arms is relaxed. The trainer then pulls back the client's arms while the client allows the stretch backwards for 15 seconds. Repeat 3 times and progress through the stretch process.

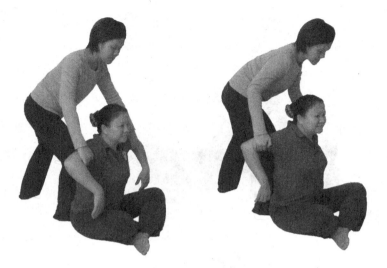

Fig. 5.1. Sequence A (left picture) and Sequence B (right picture) of the anterior deltoid and pectorals PNF muscle stretch.

Example 2: Hamstrings

❖ *Sequence A:* Using PNF technique, the trainer supports the client's leg by placing the client's ankle on the shoulder. The client pushes down on the trainer's shoulder for 6-10 seconds. Make sure both knees are kept straight, while the trainer holds the other leg down.

❖ *Sequence B:* The client relaxes the push on the trainer's shoulder and allows the trainer to gently increase the stretch of the hamstrings to a new level of comfortable tension for 15 seconds. Repeat 3 times and progress through the stretch process.

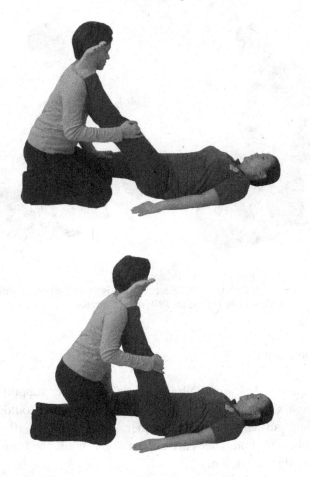

Fig. 5.2. Sequence A (top picture) and Sequence B (bottom picture) of the hamstrings PNF muscle stretch.

5.6 Other Flexibility-Based Activities and Training Aids

Yoga, Pilates and Tai Chi have gained increasing popularity in many fitness programmes in recent years. Although these programmes do not specifically focus on flexibility, they do incorporate some elements of flexibility training that can bring about improved range of motion in individual body segments and a strengthened posture. This section of the chapter briefly discusses the uniqueness of these exercise programmes and the flexibility benefits that can be derived from participation.

5.6.1 *About Yoga*

Today, Yoga has been popularised in its contemporary form, emphasising a balance between mental and physical by engaging in static poses and concentrating on patterns of breathing, physical feelings and emotions. The word "Yoga" means "union" in Sanskrit, the language of ancient India where yoga originated. It actually refers to the union or integration of the mind, body and spirit. This is because Yoga in its origin can be traced back to its historical spiritual disciplines related to Buddhist and Hindu religious practices, which also involved the teaching of moral and yogic lifestyle behavioural practices, such as meditation.

There are at least eight branches of yoga, some of which place more of its yogic emphasis on mental and spiritual well being, while few others focus more on its mental and physical components. It is important for those who are new to yoga to actively find out more and differentiate the health intents of the different branches of yoga offered in the market, and to examine own exercise needs and goals before embarking on any yoga programme.

Learning how to do basic poses correctly and developing whole body strength and flexibility are important for beginners. Beginners' poses typically include standing, seated and supine stretches, as well as simple balancing and backbend poses. At the intermediate level, as the body becomes stronger and more flexible, participants usually work on refining the basic poses and perform more difficult variations. Poses of deep backbends, intense arm balances and inversions, all of which require high degree of strength, flexibility and balance are performed at the advanced level, usually achieved through years of practice.

While performance and holding of desired poses or postures, the body is subjected to varying degrees of stretch, developing flexibility and strength at the same time. The strengthening component of the yogic exercises involve supporting the body weight in poses or postures, such as balancing on one leg, or supporting a pose with the arms. Moving slowly in and out of poses will also increase strength to the working muscles and improve overall muscle tone. In maintaining a yogic pose, the participant will be required to make small and subtle movements to improve body alignment in that particular pose, which will lead to an increased kinaesthetic awareness of own body and improved posture over time.

5.6.2 *About Pilates*

Pilates is an exercise programme developed by Joseph H. Pilates in early 1920s with a unique mental-physical emphasis, combining the science of mental focus and breathing techniques derived from Chinese martial arts and yoga with western sports science and fitness movements. Although yoga and pilates are similar in their 'mind-body' emphasis, Pilates, however, does not originate from a spiritual background.

Key principles that guide pilates workout include breathing, mental concentration, centering, control, flow and rhythm, precision, and relaxation - all of which work together in tandem and, when properly applied, produce positive physiological and psychological health benefits.

Pilates exercise movements, performed with or without the use of resistance equipment, are described as low-impact and slow with control and form. Exercises performed using a resistance-based machine, called a Reformer, can be done in various postures such as lying down, sitting, kneeling or standing. Pilates exercises aim to strengthen the core muscles that provide support for the spine and keep the body balanced.

Although Pilates is not targeted to specifically work on flexibility, it incorporates elements of flexibility training in its exercise regime. The increases of flexibility in individual body segments are primarily gained from the ballistic movements used to increase strength.

As Pilates workout routines are mainly gentle and low impact that aim to strengthen the back and spine, participants can expect increase strength and general toning of core muscles without developing much muscle bulk. Learning proper breathing and performing, or relearning, correct spinal and pelvic alignment can result in better kinaesthetic awareness of the body.

Pilates workouts can be customized to suit beginners and different levels of competency, starting with the fundamentals before moving on to mat work and reformer machines. It is important that beginners engage at an individual comfort level and seek proper instruction and supervision.

5.6.3 *About Tai Chi*

Tai Chi, also called Tai Chi Chuan, which has its origin from China deriving from a martial arts background, is a non-competitive exercise programme comprising of seemingly relaxed and gentle physical movements and stretching.

Today, Tai Chi is perhaps one of the most popular exercise programmes among men and women in the middle and elderly age groups in Singapore. Because of its self-paced nature, Tai Chi as an exercise programme is suitable for anyone, regardless of age or physical ability.

There are variations to the forms or styles of Tai Chi, and the intensity of the exercise programme will depend on the choice of the form or style practiced. Some are fast-paced while most forms are gentle in movements.

Tai Chi movements come in rhythmic patterns that are coordinated with breathing, and thus it proposes to promote wellness of the body and mind through the sequence of the Tai Chi movements which requires a person's calm concentration and production of movements flowing smoothly into each other.

5.6.4 *Stability exercises*

The stability ball is also known as a Fit Ball, gym ball, Swiss ball or flexibility ball. It is made of rubber materials, large and inflated. It is based on the principle of creating instability or resistance which requires the person to make use of the core muscles to attain balance while performing the exercise.

Using the stability ball to perform strength or flexibility exercises, or used in combination with crunches, curls, or stretching exercises, will subject the body to adapt to unusual positions and allow the recruitment of many stabilizing muscles to aid the enhancement of overall flexibility, muscular strength and endurance.

In the past, physical therapists originally used stability balls with patients suffering from spinal injuries or neurological damages as a low impact rehabilitation tool for increasing flexibility and strength. Today, stability balls are commonly found in almost every gym and fitness training centre.

Stability balls are inexpensive and, interestingly, can also be used outside of exercise workout programme if the client is creative. For instance, sitting on a stability ball instead of a desk chair will keep the core muscles working while writing or typing. This can help to improve posture and avoid common injuries that take place from excessive sitting and poor posture. When choosing a stability ball, make sure it's the right size for the client's height. There are also burst-resistant balls that can hold up to 600 or more pounds suitable for overweight or obese individuals.

In flexibility training, stability balls make it easy to move from one stretch to the next, and provide a natural support for the body. As the client moves into proper alignment, core muscles in the abdomen and around the spine are engaged. Usually, muscles in the pelvic, hip, upper and lower body regions are also mobilised. Neuromuscular coordination also can be improved.

Other than using stability ball for flexibility training programme, its usage can easily be adapted into any strength training programme. Exercises with the stability ball ought to be performed at a slow, even tempo with proper instruction and supervision.

When choosing a size that is proper for the client, make sure that your client is able to sit on the ball with his or her knees and hip at 90 degrees. For those with knee problems, the hips can be slightly higher than the knees and the posture remains comfortable.

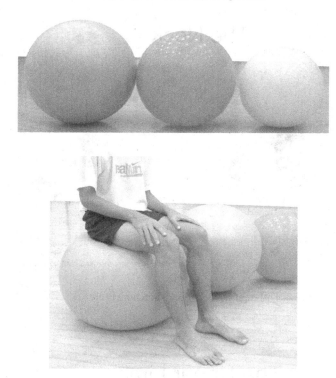

Fig. 5.3. Stability balls come in different sizes (top picture) and choosing the correct ball is important (bottom picture).

5.7 Common Flexibility and Stretching Exercises

The figures below show some of the most common flexibility and stretching exercises of the upper, lower and core body that work on muscles or muscle groups involved in various daily movements.

Remember that regular stretching of these common muscles or muscle groups can bring about many health and wellness benefits as mentioned in the earlier sections of this chapter. Even if the client is too busy for, or just not interested in, any other type of exercise programme, a simple flexibility programme is still able to provide some minimal, if not more, health benefits.

The Neck

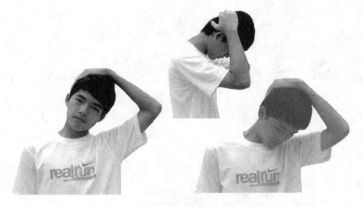

Fig. 5.4. Different types of neck stretching exercises.

The Upper Limb

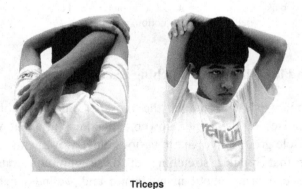

Triceps

Fig. 5.5. Upper limb – triceps stretching exercise.

The Upper Limb

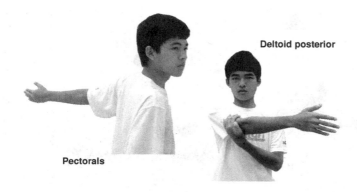

Fig. 5.6. Upper limb – pectorals and deltoid posterior stretching exercises.

The Upper Limb

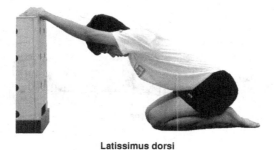

Fig. 5.7. Upper limb – latissimus dorsi stretching exercise.

The Lower Limb

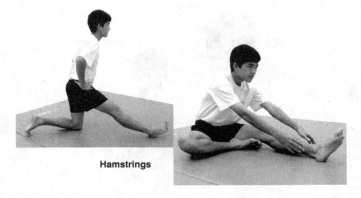

Fig. 5.8. Lower limb – hamstrings stretching exercises.

The Lower Limb

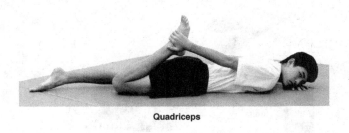

Fig. 5.9. Lower limb – quadriceps stretching exercise.

The Lower Limb

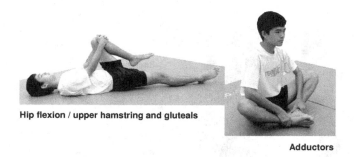

Hip flexion / upper hamstring and gluteals

Adductors

Fig. 5.10. Lower limb – upper hamstrings, gluteals, adductors stretching exercises.

The Lower Limb

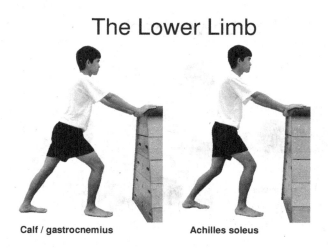

Calf / gastrocnemius   **Achilles soleus**

Fig. 5.11. Lower limb – calf/gastrocnemius, achilles soleus stretching exercises.

The Lower Back

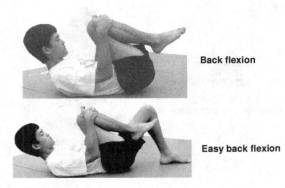

Back flexion

Easy back flexion

Fig. 5.12. Lower back – two versions of back flexion stretching exercises.

The Lower Back

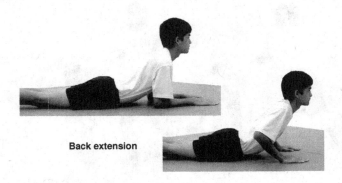

Back extension

Fig. 5.13. Lower back - two versions of back extension stretching exercises.

The Lower Back

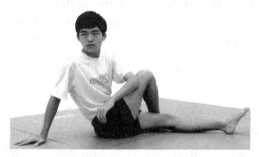

Piriformis and lower back rotation

Fig. 5.14. Lower back – piriformis and lower back rotation stretching exercise.

The Lower Back

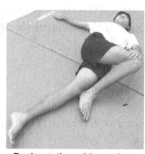 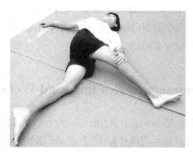

Back rotation with one leg   **Back rotation with straight leg**

Fig. 5.15. Lower back – two versions of back rotation stretching exercises.

5.8   Action Strategies

Observe common daily and sporting movements of the body. Figure out what muscles or muscle groups are involved in the production of these movements, and the specific stretching exercises for various daily health and fitness needs (e.g., general fitness, a type of sports, or relaxation).

5.9   In the News

Check out news and magazine articles or features on flexibility exercises for health, posture, common sports, including golf. Highlight interest groups and benefits that can be derived.

5.10   Summary and Key Points

There are many health benefits that can be gained from a well-balanced flexibility training programme, regardless of entry point or age. Apart from gaining the understanding of how flexibility can positively enhance general lifestyle, functional health and wellness in our daily lives, the purposeful discussions of issues pertaining to flexibility training methods, proper stretching techniques, as well as stretching activities provided in this chapter aim to provide a safe and effective guide to trainers who wish to help their clients embark on a meaningful flexibility training journey today.

5.11   Recommended Readings and Website Resource

(1) *ACSM's Resource Manual for Guidelines for Exercise Testing and Prescription* (2001). 4th Ed. ACSM, USA.
(2) Alter, M.J. (1996). *Science of Flexibility*. Human Kinetics, USA.
(3) Chia, M., Leong, L.L. and Quek, J.J. (2004). *Healthy, Well and Wise: Take PRIDE for a Life of Wellness*. National Institute of Education, Singapore. Order details: Office of Graduate Programmes and Professional Learning.

(4) Rush, A.K. (1997). *The Modern Book of Stretching: Strength and Flexibility at Any Age*. Dell Publishing, New York.

(5) Developed by a team of sport specialists from the National Institute of Education, SSSS is a scientific and holistic approach to understanding and practising the principles of science for conditioning for health and fitness. SSSS will help clients get the most out of their sporting pursuits, training, practice or competition: www.sportsuccess.nie.edu.sg.

(6) http://www.mayoclinic.com is an award-winning consumer Web site that offers health information, self-improvement and disease management tools. This website contains relevant health and fitness related resources such as healthy living articles, videos and slide shows that fitness professionals will find useful.

Chapter 6

Designing Strength and Endurance Resistance Programmes

Strength and endurance resistance conditioning can be conducted using body weight, machines and free weights. Specific forms of resistance conditioning exercises require special attention to proper alignment, proper posture, and proper speed of execution, proper breathing techniques and proper stretching exercises. Strength and resistance training programmes adhere to the same general principles of training.

After completing this chapter, you will be able to:

- ❖ Understand the functions of different types of weight training machines - isoinertial and isokinetic machines.
- ❖ Plan a holistic progressive resistance training programme for a client who is interested in general condition for muscular strength and muscular endurance, for muscular endurance and for muscular strength.
- ❖ Be conversant with the equivalent weight training exercises using free weights - dumbbells, barbells and body weight.

6.1 Introduction

Personal trainers must be familiar with different methods of resistance training using machines, free weights and body weight. Different types of resistance training exercises using state-of-the-art weight training machines are available. Most machines are isoinertial resistance machines while some rehabilitative machines are isokinetic in nature.

6.2   Different Methods of Resistance Training

Free weight exercises, using dumbbells and barbells provide a greater range of motion than machines and more variety of motion but are more difficult to control to maintain good form and posture and body alignment in performing the exercise, especially for beginners.

Table 6.1. Considerations for using isoinertial machines.

Characteristics	Advantages	Disadvantages	Remarks
Fixed inertia mass, variable resistance through range of motion, exercise done at variable velocity.	Customised for adult posture and adjustable for different sizes. Body alignment is usually controlled for. Exercise guided through fixed range of motion.	Limited range of motion that may not mimic movement in sport.	Good start for beginners as there are less safety concerns.

Table 6.2. Considerations for using isokinetic machines.

Characteristics	Advantages	Disadvantages	Remarks
Fixed velocity of movement as resistance is increased with the speed of motion.	Effective for rehabilitative purposes.	Does not mimic sport performance as the velocity of motion is controlled and is externally not very motivating. No visual feedback about the amount of resistance being used motivating.	For beginners who wish to get a feel for resistance exercise without any visual feedback about the amount of resistance used.

Table 6.3. Considerations for using body weight.

Characteristics	Advantages	Disadvantages	Remarks
Using the body weight of body parts and segments to provide resistance.	No equipment is necessary. By adopting certain body posture and pivot points, different degrees of difficulty can be adjusted.	Resistance offered by different body parts or segments are fixed- may be too light or too heavy. Does not allow for very much variety.	May not be motivating for beginners especially when muscle strength and endurance are weak.

However, incorporating machines and free weight resistance exercises provide the client with variety and allow for more programming options. It is important to take client interest and preference into consideration when selecting the mode of resistance exercises for the client.

Table 6.4. Considerations for using free weights.

Characteristics	Advantages	Disadvantages	Remarks
Dumbells and barbells. Also isoinertial masses used.	Greater variety and flexibility in performing the exercise with a greater range of motion and body posture.	Less control in terms of body posture and alignment in performing the exercise. Must exercise greater care and concern regarding safety of use- e.g. use of weight collars.	Useful as a progression from weight machines. Provides variety for performing exercises. Need to exercise greater attention to body posture, body alignment, range of motion and speed of performing the exercise.

Always perform large muscle group cardiovascular exercises like brisk-walking, jogging, rowing or cycling at a client determined pace for about 10 minutes to raise core muscle temperature, before embarking on resistance training.

Table 6.5. Considerations for using resistance bands.

Characteristics	Advantages	Disadvantages	Remarks
Colour-coded in terms of the degree of resistance that they provide.	Affordable and portable so can be used at home and in the office for a simple workout.	Care that the band is held in a firm grip, otherwise it may become elastic nature of the band may hit and hurt someone nearby. The band can only offer minimal overload in terms of resistance.	The elastic band can provide for a wide variety of exercises using just the different body parts. Clients must be taught the proper way of performing each exercise for effectiveness.

6.3 Conducting the Workout: Essential Knowledge and Sequence

Typical know-how of resistance training for personal trainers include: name of the machine, name of the exercise, the major muscles exercised, the proper form, technique, body posture and body alignment, speed and repetitions for performing the exercise and the associated muscle stretch after performing the exercise.

For beginners, incorporate large-muscle group and whole body conditioning and build up muscle endurance first, before progressing to training for muscular strength. Time should be set aside for core muscle conditioning as these would help with energy transfer of the muscles when the spine, shoulder and hip girdles are stabilised.

6.3.1 *Name of the machine*

This is usually named after the major muscle groups that the exercise targets and the action of the exercise- e.g. Lat pull-down machine- the primary muscle group used is the latissimus dorsi and the exercise action is a pull-down with both arms, placed at shoulder-width apart. Personal trainers must check the condition of the machine, associated cables, pulleys, moving parts and upholstery to ensure that they are in good working condition.

6.3.2 *Name of the muscle groups used*

Machines typically work multi-muscle groups. In the case of the Lat Pull-Down machine, the muscle groups worked are the latissimus dorsi, the deltoids, the triceps and the biceps.

6.3.3 *Proper body posture and alignment*

It is important that personal trainers pay careful attention to the correct body posture and body alignment in relation to the exercise. This means checking on the position of the body joints of neck, shoulder, elbows, wrist, hip, knees, and ankles before and throughout the exercise.

Reinforce good posture and make sure that the vulnerable body parts (neck and lower back) are always supported. Additionally, where possible avoid body posture that raises blood pressure- overhead presses, decline presses, etc unnecessarily or exercises with a high cost-benefit ratio (i.e. risk of the exercise is less than the benefit of performing the exercise).

6.3.4 *Perform a safe range of motion*

Ensure that there is a safe range of motion for performing the exercise. Keep joints flexed and not locked at the end of performing the exercise so that the joints do not bear the brunt of shock absorption of performing the exercise.

6.3.5 *Perform a controlled speed of motion*

Personal trainers should ensure that the clients perform each exercise in a controlled speed (count of 1000, 2000), and master the speed and rhythm of performing the exercise.

6.3.6 *Breathing*

Clients must never hold their breath whilst performing any resistance training exercises. Personal trainers must cue clients to breathe out on effort (active part of the exercise) and breathe in on the passive part of the exercise. When in doubt, personal trainers should just cue the client to breathe normally. Breath-holding during resistance training may cause the client to 'black out'.

6.3.7 *Reinforce good form of performing each exercise*

For the personal trainer, this means checking on the proper body posture and body alignment, speed and range of motion and breathing of the client when he/she is performing the exercise. Check with the client at the end of the exercise, that he/she feels the muscles being exercised are the correct ones. Personal trainers should instruct the client to focus and concentrate on performing each exercise in good form.

6.3.8 *Perform specific stretching after the set*

At the end of each set, personal trainers should guide the client through a specific muscle stretch for the major muscle group that was exercised. Check stretching posture and body alignment of the stretch, easing the stretch by breathing out and stretch to point of mild discomfort, hold the stretch for at least 10 seconds and breathe normally. Relax and repeat the stretch again where necessary.

6.3.9 *Plan for muscle balance*

Perform exercises for each of the major muscle groups- back, shoulders and chest, front and back of the arm, abdominals and lower back, front and back of the thigh, and calves. A circuit of 8-10 exercise stations is a good start for beginners. Perform a set of 10-15 repetitions (training equally for muscular strength and muscular endurance), with a recovery interval of between 1-3 minutes to allow for adequate recovery between sets. Each set should leave the client close to fatigue but adjustments and refinements may be necessary so that straining whilst performing each exercise is kept to a minimum.

6.3.10 *Core muscle conditioning*

Core muscle conditioning is essential for maintaining pain-free lower back health and for sport performance. The muscles that support the spine, hip and shoulder girdles must be targeted. These muscles stabilize the spine, and trunk so that forces are appropriately transferred when muscles contract. Body weight exercises such as push-ups, V-sit ups, lunges, back extensions, hip lifts and squats as well as yoga and Pilates are good exercise forms for core muscle conditioning. Muscles that should be targeted for core muscle conditioning include the abdominals, erector spinae, gluteal and hip flexor and adductus muscles.

6.3.11 *Reduce delayed onset of muscle soreness*

This can be done by selecting lighter resistance (load) and increasing the number of repetitions per set, and allowing a longer recovery period (e.g. 5 minutes) before performing the same set of exercise.

6.4 Training for Muscular Endurance and Muscular Strength

For beginners to resistance training, always train for muscular endurance before muscular strength. There needs to be some trial and error in deciding with each client, the actual resistance to select for each exercise. As a guide, the resistance selected should result in near fatigue when performing the final repetition.

Table 6.6. General information for muscular endurance and strength fitness training.

Fitness type	Number of repetitions per set	Remarks
Muscle endurance	16-25	Fatigue at 25 rep
Muscle strength	6 or less	Fatigue at 6 or less rep
Muscle endurance and strength	10-15	Fatigue at 15 rep

6.5 Sample Resistance Training Exercises

6.5.1 *Useful tips to start out on resistance training*

- ❖ Always warm-up first.
- ❖ Check that machine is in good and safe working order.
- ❖ When using barbell and dumbell, always secure the collars.
- ❖ Adjust machine for body size and exercise load.
- ❖ Perform multi-muscle group exercises.
- ❖ Ensure good body posture and alignment.
- ❖ Breathe out on effort and breathe in on the passive phase.
- ❖ Perform the full safe range of motion.
- ❖ Regulate the speed as counting 1000, 2000.
- ❖ Train for muscle balance.

❖ Develop muscular endurance first before muscular strength.
❖ Concentrate on performing each exercise in good form and technique.
❖ Use machines, free weights or body weight to inject variety into the workout.

6.5.2 *Exercises using machines*

❖ Take note of machine features.
❖ Ensure proper posture.
❖ Ensure proper alignment.
❖ Perform exercise in good form and in a controlled manner.

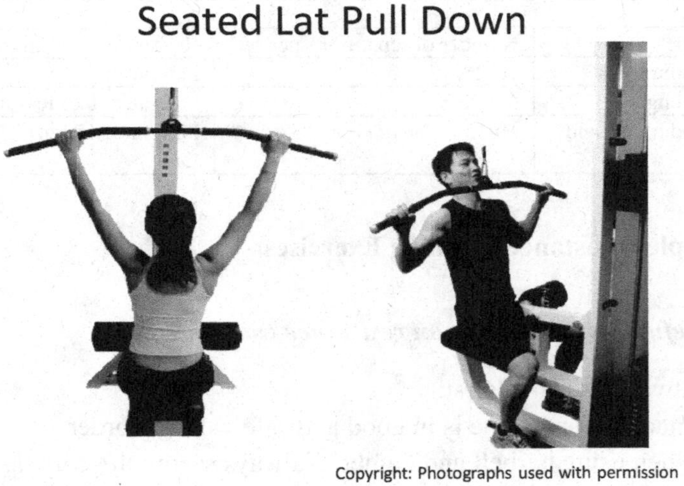

Seated Lat Pull Down

Copyright: Photographs used with permission

Fig. 6.1. Exercises using machines – seated lat pull down.

Seated Chest Press

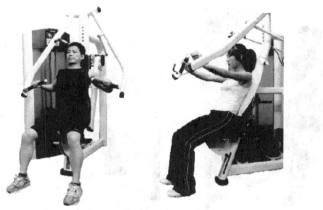

Copyright: Photographs used with permission

Fig. 6.2. Exercises using machines – seated chest press.

Seated Deltoid Raise

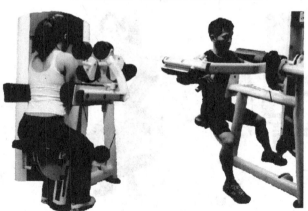

Copyright: Photographs used with permission

Fig. 6.3. Exercises using machines – seated deltoid raise.

Seated Shoulder Pull

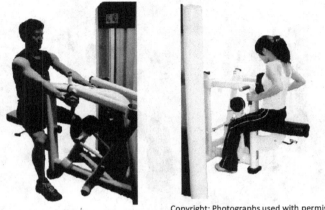

Fig. 6.4. Exercises using machines – seated shoulder pull.

Seated Bicep Curl

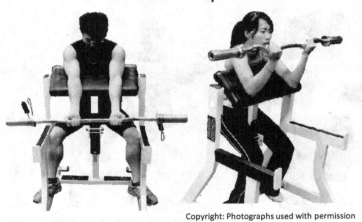

Fig. 6.5. Exercises using machines – seated biceps curl.

Standing Tricep Extension

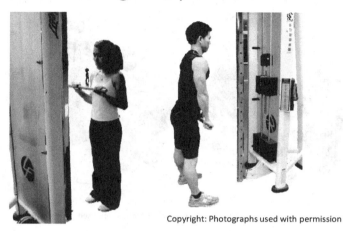

Copyright: Photographs used with permission

Fig. 6.6. Exercises using machines – standing tricep extension.

Seated Leg Press

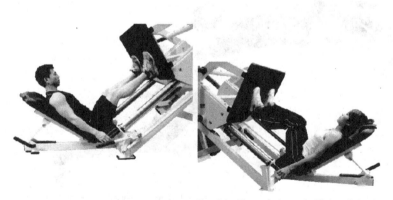

Copyright: Photographs used with permission

Fig. 6.7. Exercises using machines – seated leg press.

Supine Leg Curl

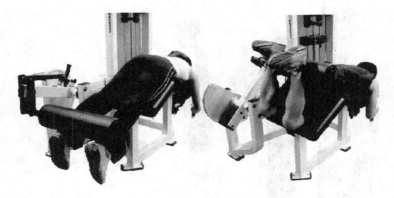

Copyright: Photographs used with permission

Fig. 6.8. Exercises using machines – supine leg curl.

Inclined Curl Up

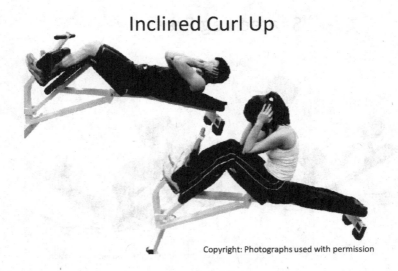

Copyright: Photographs used with permission

Fig. 6.9. Exercises using machines – inclined curl up.

Lower Back Extension

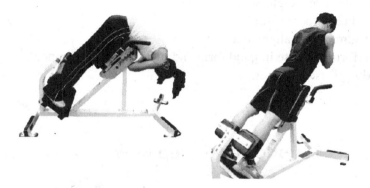

Copyright: Photographs used with permission

Fig. 6.10. Exercises using machines – lower back extension.

Hip Flex

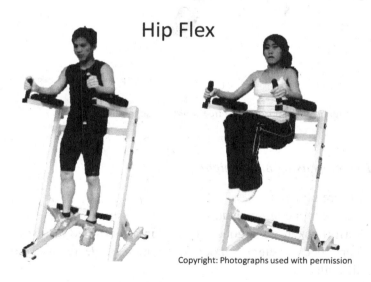

Copyright: Photographs used with permission

Fig. 6.11. Exercises using machines – hip flex.

6.5.3　*Exercises using free weight*

- ❖ Always use weight collars.
- ❖ Ensure proper posture.
- ❖ Ensure proper alignment.
- ❖ Perform exercise in good form and in a controlled manner.
- ❖ Always use a spotter.

Supported Tricep Row

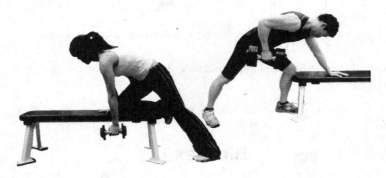

Copyright: Photographs used with permission

Fig. 6.12. Exercises using free weights – supported tricep row.

6.5.4　*Exercises using body weight*

- ❖ Ensure proper posture.
- ❖ Ensure proper alignment.
- ❖ Perform exercise in good form and in a controlled manner.
- ❖ Vary body weight supported to increase/decrease degree of difficulty.

Push up

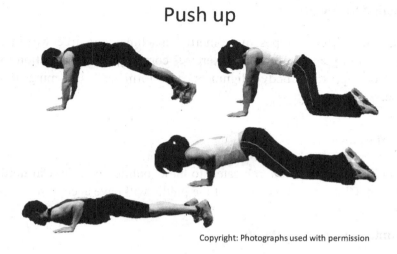

Fig. 6.13. Exercises using body weight – push up.

Pull Up

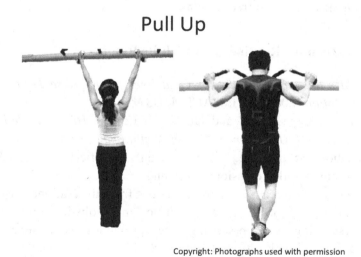

Fig. 6.14. Exercises using body weight – pull up.

6.6 Action Strategies

Practise with different types of isoinertial machines and free weights. Always warm-up and perform the exercises correctly paying attention to proper body posture, body alignment and form of performing the exercise.

6.7 In the News

Body building association relocates to new public gym in Cairnhill Community Club, where members of the public will have access to.

6.8 Summary and Key Points

Isoinertial machines, isokinetic machines, and free weights can be used for progressive resistance training for muscular strength and endurance. Personal trainers should practise good safety, establish a routine for taking a client through a training circuit and practice good gym habits when using machines and free weights.

6.9 Recommended Readings and Website Resource

(1) *ACSM's Resource Manual for Guidelines for Exercise Testing and Prescription* (2001). 4th Ed. ACSM, USA.

(2) Chia, M., Leong, L.L. and Quek, J.J. (2004). *Healthy, Well and Wise: Take PRIDE for a Life of Wellness.* National Institute of Education, Singapore. Order details: Office of Graduate Programmes and Professional Learning.

(3) Developed by a team of sport specialists from the National Institute of Education, SSSS is a scientific and holistic approach to understanding and practising the principles of science for conditioning for health and fitness. SSSS will help clients get the most out of their sporting pursuits, training, practice or competition: www.sportsuccess.nie.edu.sg

Chapter 7

Designing the Cardiovascular Programme

Having sufficient cardiovascular fitness is necessary to carry out everyday tasks and recreation without undue fatigue, but with some measures of ease and enjoyment. Training for cardiovascular fitness does not have to be boring or repetitive. It is an art, as much as it is a science, to be able to plan out a series of fun, motivating and effective exercise or physical activity regimens that can enhance your client's cardiovascular fitness, which in turn can improve his or her quality of life.

After completing this chapter, you will be able to:

❖ Understand basic principles of cardiorespiratory system and the energy systems.

❖ Know and apply principles of training for cardiovascular fitness requirements.

❖ Able to design, plan, and instruct cardiovascular training programmes.

7.1 Introduction

Many people understand the benefits of having the different aspects of physical fitness, such as strength, endurance, power, speed, flexibility and agility in relation to sports and specialized training.

Some people mistakenly think that endurance is only an ability of athletes who participate in long-distance events. There are also many who still do not know the benefits of having adequate cardiovascular fitness, or aerobic fitness, in daily life for non-sporting population.

The body systems used in physical activities and exercise, for instance the heart, lungs and muscles become stronger and fitter over time. Regular participation in physical activities and exercises following sound principles of training causes the body systems to adapt.

What this means is that the more often one exercises or trains, provided without subjecting to overtraining, the more adapted or fitter the body becomes.

Truly in sports, having a good endurance foundation can increase an athlete's ability to stay on the task or event for as long as possible without slowing down too much or becoming tired too soon. In the same way, individuals with a good or sufficient level of aerobic fitness tend to cope better with work and other aspects of their lifestyles more easily.

In the context of personal training, the role of personal trainer extends to helping clients achieve functional aerobic fitness not just to achieve specific physical gains, but also to achieve improved ability to enjoy work and leisure in daily living.

It is important that trainers understand sound principles of cardiovascular training and how to choose exercise activities that clients are likely to enjoy in the course of personal training. The principles and concepts of planning and designing good cardiovascular training programmes are discussed in this chapter.

7.2 Basic Principles of the Energy Systems

All human beings rely on our energy systems to live and to play. We briefly learned in Chapter 4 that the energy system help us to convert the energy from food into useful muscle energy for bodily movement during training and exercise, and that appropriate training can help fine-tune the energy system components.

Adenosine triphospate (ATP) is the body's energy source to drive muscle contractions and perform other bodily functions and is supplied via the energy system both aerobically and anaerobically.

The energy system and its component characteristics are described in Tables 7.1 to 7.3 below (adapted and modified from Sports Science in Sporting Success by Chia et al., 2007 with permission).

Table 7.1. Characteristics of the ATP-CP system.

> ❖ Energy in the form of ATP is provided without the need for oxygen (i.e. it is anaerobic).
>
> ❖ Natural amounts of creatine phosphate (CP), also known as phosphocreatine, are found within the muscle and a main source of creatine is from meat.
>
> ❖ The energy is provided almost instantaneously but at this very fast speed, the energy can only last about 20-30 seconds of all out effort exercise e.g. sprinting over 100-200m, doing a fast break in basketball or running down the sidelines with the ball in soccer or hockey or rugby.
>
> ❖ The energy is replaced in the presence of oxygen during the recovery period (i.e. breathing very hard and fast after a sprint and walking slowly) in about 3 minutes. About 50% of the energy used is replaced in about 30 seconds.
>
> ❖ Specific training can help an athlete improve energy supply and also faster recovery in energy supply.

Table 7.2. Characteristics of the Lactic Acid system.

> ❖ The energy is also provided without the need for oxygen (i.e. it is also anaerobic).
>
> ❖ The natural source of energy comes from muscle glycogen or stored carbohydrate in the muscle.
>
> ❖ In terms of speed, the energy is provided swiftly but its speed in providing energy is only 50% that of the ATP-CP system. However, it has 200% of the capacity of energy of the ATP-CP system.
>
> ❖ In activities that are intense and last up to 2 minutes or less, the lactic acid system plays an important role. Examples of activities that are powered by the lactic acid system include sprinting, throwing, jumping, rowing and swimming activities at intense exercise levels.
>
> ❖ However, in using this energy system, lactic acid will eventually accumulate within the muscles resulting in fatigue.
>
> ❖ Specific training can help better utilisation of this energy system and also a greater tolerance of the physical discomforts of lactic acid accumulation.

It is not true that the energy system works independently of each other. All components of the energy system work together in an integrated manner. For example, for a 10km running event, the aerobic energy system predominates up to 80%, while the anaerobic systems contribute the remaining 20% to the energy production. The extent of energy supply from the aerobic and anaerobic energy systems will depend on mainly on how intense the exercise is and how long the exercise lasts.

Table 7.3. Characteristics of the Oxygen Energy system.

> ❖ Also known as the Aerobic Energy System. Aerobic means "with oxygen". This component of the energy system, as the name implies requires oxygen for energy supply.
>
> ❖ This energy system can supply energy for low to moderate intensity exercise for long periods of time.
>
> ❖ Its main energy source is from fatty acids (i.e. fat), glucose (i.e. carbohydrate) and amino acids (i.e. protein). However, proteins do not play a major role in contributing energy for exercise.
>
> ❖ This energy system provides the main source of energy especially for activities at rest and also during exercise of a low to moderate intensity lasting 3 minutes or more and also during the recovery periods between sprints in team sports like hockey, netball, soccer and rugby.

When the exercise intensity is low, the energy needs of the body can be met by mainly by the oxygen energy system. However as the exercise intensity increases, there will be increased contribution to the energy supply from the lactic acid system and when the intensity increases to maximal effort, there will also be energy contribution from the ATP-CP system. During 'start and go' type of exercise activities, there is a great deal of overlap in energy supply from both aerobic and anaerobic sources.

For most people, when the exercise last less than 30s, the effort is all out, and the energy is provided mainly by the ATP-CP system (anaerobic). For exercise lasting between 30s and 3 minutes, the exercise effort can be said to be intense and the energy is provided mainly by the lactic acid system. For an exercise greater than 3 minutes, the exercise effort can be described as low to moderate, the energy is provided mainly by the oxygen system.

In the context of personal training, training for cardiovascular fitness focuses on the training of the oxygen-delivery and aerobic metabolism mechanisms of the Oxygen Energy System. Most cells in the body rely on a constant supply of oxygen and nutrients via the bloodstreams to these cells for the production of energy necessary for cellular and other bodily functions.

Training the *cardiorespiratory* system (is also known as the *cardiovascular system* as expressed in many textbooks) deals with conditioning and improving the ability of the heart and blood circulation through a vast network of blood vessels and capillaries (*cardio*), as well as the lungs and the exchange of gases (*respiratory*). The exchange of gases not only occurs at the lungs, but also at the capillaries through the peripheral tissues of the body. Briefly, by-products of energy metabolism, such as lactic acid and carbon dioxide, are removed from the cells into the bloodstream. The former, which can be converted back as a useful fuel is further metabolised and oxidized for energy production, is carried to the liver while the latter is carried to the lungs for disposal.

7.3 Principles of Training and Programming Adapting to Client's Needs

Personal trainers need to accept that not all clients have the same level of fitness, motor abilities, personal characteristics and psychological attributes. Coming from different backgrounds, cultures, having different lifestyles, previous exercise or training experiences, as well as education levels do make a difference in client's needs and exercise goals. Other differences, particularly seen in older individuals, could evolve around work schedules, financial and family commitments, etc.

It is not so much about the trainer having the knowledge of the principle of training to help the clients improve in aerobic fitness, it is more important that the trainer, having good understanding of the principle of training, is able to adjust and cater training programmes to suit the individual capabilities, needs and preferences for physical fitness and wellness.

7.3.1 *General guidelines apply*

Generally, the guidelines for designing safe and effective cardiovascular exercise programme for most of the population are expressed in the table below:

Table 7.4. General guidelines for designing cardiovascular exercise programme.

Frequency	Three to five sessions per week.
Intensity	Between 60-90% of maximum heart rate. Other more sensitive formulas for determining exercise intensity for aerobic conditioning will be discussed in greater details in the latter part of this chapter.
Duration	20-60 minutes per session. Discontinuous or intermittent bouts of at least 10 minutes can also total up to 20 to 60 minutes.
Type	Aerobic type exercise such as brisk-walking, jogging, swimming or cycling. Other types of aerobic exercise activities are discussed in more details in the latter part of this chapter.

Of course, for beginners, they should start at the lower end of the prescription (3 days per week, 20 minutes per session, and exercising at 60% of max HR) and gradually build up. Moderate to vigorous exercise is suitable and recommended for most individuals.

For overweight, deconditioned or unfit individuals who are starting an exercise programme after a long-term sedentary lifestyle, it is advisable to embark on a shorter duration ˈlower-intensity exercise activity. For those who are interested in improving general cardiovascular health, three times per week for at least 20 per session may be sufficient.

To improve aerobic fitness, depending on the current entry level, three to four times a week for at least 30 minutes per session will yield reasonable results. Regardless what the exercise goals are, obtain medical clearance before embarking on any serious training programme.

7.3.2 *Improving aerobic fitness and optimising gains*

A brief overview of the principle of training suitable for any training programme is provided in an earlier chapter. In this chapter, we will be elaborating a little more below on how some of these principles of training can be applied in planning cardiovascular training programme to produce the most optimal aerobic fitness gain for each unique client.

All training responses are the result of stress and adaptation. This means there must be exposure over a period of time in terms of an appropriate amount of exercise effort, beyond that to which it is accustomed to, in order for the body to be fitter and stronger.

Safe overload exposures are within 10-30% of what is accustomed by the client on a daily basis. For improvements in fitness, there must be progressions in overload. These progressions should be advanced only when the client is accustomed to the overload. This usually takes about 4 to 6 weeks. A one-size-fits-all exercise programme should not be used for all clients.

The recommended rate of progression of overload exposure varies with individual. For example, for overweight, deconditioned or unfit individuals who are starting an exercise programme after a long-term sedentary lifestyle, in such cases, an even smaller progression of overload exposures just within 5 to 10% for 4 to 6 weeks are advisable. Hence it is important to personalize and individualize the exercise programme to suit each client.

In any training programme, the trainer can increase the training load progressively and appropriately and apply sound reasoning in exercise programming in the following areas:

7.3.2.1 *Increase the duration of training sessions*

The duration of each training session can be gradually increased from the beginning of the training programme. For example, at the start of the programme, each session may only last 30 minutes, but eventually, the duration for training may extend as long as 1 hr 30 min towards the end of the programme.

Some of the approaches a trainer might consider as the duration of the training session increase could be:

- ❖ Incorporate a variety of activities to keep up the client's interest.
- ❖ Have longer or adequate rest between activities.
- ❖ Consider if the weather is too hot and humid for a long session.
- ❖ Consider whether the activities could be conducted indoor or outdoor for variation.
- ❖ Consider heat illness and hydration issues.

7.3.2.2 *Increase the number of exercises/drills per session*

Trainers can slowly introduce and implement more and varied exercises, activities, drills and repetitions over the weeks and months. However, it is important to remember the need to monitor the client closely, and whether there is sufficient rest and recovery as the number, as well as the complexity of exercises, activities, drills and repetitions increases.

Having enough rest between activities and exercises is most important to ensure that the client is able to complete most or all of the work planned for that training session.

7.3.2.3 *Increase the frequency of training sessions*

Most of the time, as your client gets fitter and stronger, there may well be a need to increase the frequency of training sessions in order to experience more improvement in fitness and motor abilities.

The frequency, or number of training sessions per week, should be progressively increased throughout the training programme, and not be abruptly introduced. However, it is better to increase the duration of the training sessions, before increasing the frequency of sessions.

For example, you might want to begin with twice a week of training for 45 minutes per session, and gradually up the duration to 1 hr 30 min still at twice a week for a period of time before increasing to three times a week. This will allow the client to gradually build up his or her tolerance for training as well.

7.3.2.4 *More is not always better*

Here is an important fact to keep in mind – more is not always better! Trainers and clients should understand that fitness improvements are the summation of the physiological adaptations induced by regular exercise. This requires an optimum frequency of training sessions repeated regularly for the duration of the training programme.

Two important factors should be kept in mind. Firstly, the adaptation is specific to the stress, and secondly, all adaptation takes place during recovery. Rest and recovery are also essential for the body to get rid of exercise metabolites and for the body to replenish muscle nutrients and for the body to repair bodily wear and tear.

Here are some useful pointers to remember:

- ❖ In general, a recovery period of 48 to 72 hours between exercise sessions may be required.
- ❖ Closely spaced long sessions of exercise workouts should be avoided.
- ❖ Alternate easy and more intense workouts during a training week for proper recovery.
- ❖ The intensity, frequency and duration of workouts must match the capabilities of the client, and not always about what the trainer thinks is best.

7.3.2.5 *Know what is "failing adaptation"*

Because not all clients have the same tolerance to training, when a client presents symptoms of prolonged fatigue, the trainer ought to adjust the training programme and allow adequate recovery for this particular client. Be sensitive to how the client feels throughout the training programme. Excessive training programmes that overload the client with insufficient recovery will lead to breakdown and loss of performance. If the stress is too intense or too frequent, adaptation is not possible. This is often called "failing adaptation" and will result in no improvement in fitness gains and even negative improvement in performance.

Here is a list of common signs and symptoms of "failing adaptation":

❖ Increase susceptibility to coughs and colds, or falling sick often.
❖ Sleeplessness.
❖ Increase in resting heart rate of more than 10 beats per minute.
❖ Decrease skill performance.
❖ Decrease motivation level.
❖ Loss of concentration.
❖ Not eating well or losing appetite.
❖ Unexpected or drastic weight loss.
❖ Appear tired and complain of headache, fatigue all the time.
❖ Cannot keep up with usual pace, volume or workload.

7.3.2.6 *Ways to 'keep on keeping on'*

The rates of improvement in fitness are dependent on the entry level of fitness at the beginning of the programme, usually greater for a client whose entry level of fitness is low compared to one whose fitness level is higher. Regardless of how much fitness gains there are, once the client has attained a certain level of fitness, it becomes necessary to prevent the conditioning benefits from being lost.

This principle is really about bringing across the idea "If you don't use it, you will lose it", and is often known as the "detraining" effect. Even for athletes, in the competitive season, coaches often make provisions to maintain conditioning throughout the training season or else all the hard-earned fitness will gradually decline. After few weeks of detraining, up to 30% of the endurance capacity, muscle strength, power and speed may be lost.

It may not be easy for clients who have busy working schedules to regularly exercise and sustain fitness gained from the training programme. It is therefore important for trainers to habituate clients to the routine such that it comes part of the client's schedule of life as early as possible.

At least a minimum of two quality exercise sessions of up to 45 minutes per week may be necessary to prevent fitness decline. This could mean a need to reassess training goals and introduce a variety of training by incorporating mixed or cross-training.

Mixed or cross-training involves different routines and exposures to different forms of weight resistance training (free, machines, body weight), flexibility exercises (static, PNF), and cardiovascular training (interval, continuous, fartlek) which may provide better motivation for the client. Adding variety to training sessions will prevent boredom and staleness.

Introducing new forms of exercises and activities, including sports and games, may well add new spice and enjoyment to the exercise sessions. While mixed or cross-training is often introduced to provide for balance and variety for the long haul, the gains in fitness can definitely be maintained through such approaches.

The trainer may even conduct a training session away from the usual environment or venue. Do mind in mind that some individuals cope better with heat during training while others do not. This could be due to the differences in individuals' body composition, physique and even psychological tolerance of heat and cold. In the same way, some clients may have respiratory distress and therefore will not cope well in training environment with polluted air.

While air pollution is not of dangerous levels in Singapore as opposed to some countries, it is still quite typical that Singapore does not have many natural environments and most buildings are situated very close to major roads and junctions in commercial areas and housing estates.

7.4 Estimated Energy Expenditure of Various Sports and Physical Activities

To produce optimal benefits in aerobic fitness, the intensity of aerobic physical activities must be more vigorous than the intensity of lifestyle physical activities, such as walking to and from work, climbing the stairs rather than taking the escalator or lift, working in the garden, and doing activities as part of usual daily activities.

Aerobic activities are activities that are performed at a moderately hard to vigorous intensity for relatively long periods of time without stopping. Here, it will involve the maintenance of appropriate elevation heart rate significantly for the duration of exercise.

Energy is expended in physical activity, which can be defined as any bodily movement produced by the muscles. On the other hand, exercise is deliberately planned and structured properly. Often, an exercise programme is planned and structured in ways to suit the needs of the particular individual and aims to improve or maintain certain components of fitness.

Table 7.5. Energy expenditure in kcal/kg body mass/hour (adapted and modified from Sports Science in Sporting Success by Chia et al., 2007 with permission).

3-4	Physical education classes	Normal swimming	Walking at 4-6km/hr			
5-6	Kayaking	Rowing				
7-8	Running at 7-9 km/hr	Cycling at 15-25 km/hr	Tennis	Table tennis	Volley-ball	Waterski
9-10	Running at 9-11 km/hr	Skating at 12-14 km/hr	Cycling at 25-30 km/hr	Rowing at 6km/hr		
11-12	Swimming at 3 km/hr	Running at 12-14km/hr	Badminton	Cycling at 30-35 km/hr	Shot put	Rock climbing at 3.3 km/hr
13-14	Running at 15-17 km/hr	Cycling at 35-40 km/hr	Gymnastics, judo, kayaking	Cycling uphill	Fast swim	Soccer, hockey, netball, rugby
16-18	Cycling at 40 km/hr					
18-20	Marathon running at 16.8 km/hr @ 2hr 30min pace					
21-22	Marathon running at 18.3 km/hr @ 2hr 10min pace					

Most serious exercisers are intuitively concerned about the calories expended when exercising and are curious to know if a particular exercise or physical activity is effective in expending the desired amount of calories. Being able to provide accurate estimates of the amount of calories expended would be useful and possibly help to motivate clients to take on exercise within the routines of daily life for health and weight management.

The energy used during physical activity, exercise and sporting activities will depend on the intensity and duration of the activity and also on the body mass of the person. The trainer can gauge the estimated energy expended in any aerobic exercise through the measurement of calorie expended.

This approach is useful for exercise or training programmes targeted at weight management, particularly if there is a need to monitor energy intake and expenditure. For example, if the aim is to burn 1,500 kilocalories per week, this could be divided into 3 exercise sessions of 500 kilocalories per session in that week. In the same way, the energy expenditure in mixed or cross-training exercise session can also be easily calculated.

7.4.1 *A typical guideline for most people of normal weight*

For most people of normal weight, to expend about 250 to 300 calories a day, exercise examples include up to 30 minutes of rowing machine exercise, swimming or bicycle at moderate to moderately high intensity, approximately 35 to 40 minutes of jog, up to 40 to 50 minutes of brisk walk, or approximately up to 90 minutes of normal-paced walk.

7.4.2 *Choosing the right modes of aerobic exercise activity*

Aerobic exercise is exercise that involves or improves oxygen consumption (i.e. transport and uptake of oxygen by muscles). Aerobic exercise typically uses large muscle groups in a continuous manner. There are many types of aerobic exercise, and they are performed at moderate to vigorous levels of intensity for extended periods of time. Participating in appropriate aerobic exercises on a regular basis will bring about many health benefits. These include improved mood, stress relief, improved aerobic fitness, improved blood profile, healthy blood pressure management, better sleep, higher energy turnover, and weight loss or weight maintenance.

7.5   Three Basic Phases of a Training Session

Before we go on to discuss on the types of aerobic exercise activities, it is necessary here to mention three basic phases (warm-up phase, work-out phase, cool-down phase) of an exercise session that trainers ought to implement to ensure that every session is safely administered. The three phases are as follows:

7.5.1   *Warm-up phase*

A general warm-up, which could take 5 to 15 minutes, should initiate the training session. An objective of the warm-up could be to prepare the client physically and mentally for the demand of the training session. The warm-up has the intent to raise body temperature and should involve all body components, particularly the large and deep muscles.

In the warm-up, start off gentle and raise the intensity of activities gradually. After this aspect of the warm-up, simple stretching exercises involving the major joints should be included. The stretches are usually static (still) and held to a point of slight discomfort (not pain) for between 10 and 30 seconds each. A slight elevation of heart rate is also a benefit of warm-up and stays around 50 to 60% of the target heart rate.

7.5.2   *Work-out phase*

The work out phase usually lasts from 20-60 minutes. Strenuous, high intensity workouts (i.e. interval training) may be suitable for athletes training for competitive sports, but for most of the population, such workouts are not encouraged. Most people will be comfortable with workouts of fixed steady state exercise intensity, and even some speed play incorporated into the exercise session after some time into the training programme.

Of course, there are also others who prefer more group-based or fun-based aerobic activities such as hip-hop dancing and rollerblading. More senior individuals may even prefer slightly less intense workouts such as brisk-walking or a leisure bike ride along the nature reserve treks, or ballroom dancing. Some may even prefer participating in an organized sport. There is always something for everyone!

Table 7.6. Three main types of cardiovascular conditioning for aerobic fitness.

Fixed steady state exercise intensity -- e.g. running, cycling or swimming at fixed relative exercise intensity for 20 minutes or more. Gradually progress to 30-60 minutes.
Interval training -- e.g. high intensity running for 10-15 minutes, interspersed with 10-15 minutes of low intensity walking or rest, repeated several times in the training session.
Speed play or fartlek -- e.g. Speed of running is varied at different stages or durations depending on how the client feels on the day. Slope or gradient of running can be used to vary the pace.

7.5.3 Cool-down phase

At the end of the training session, the client performs the cool-down to gradually bring the body function back to normal levels. An abrupt stop to the aerobic work-out is not ideal and is considered unsafe. Like the warm-up phase, the he cool down phase may take 5-15 minutes. Cooling down activities can include light, general exercises such as slow walking, and simple general stretching, again involving the major joints.

7.6 Common Cardiovascular Activities

Most types of aerobic exercise mentioned below will suit any age group. These aerobic exercises do not require complicated machines or gym equipment. Most can be performed in the outdoor. Other than having a good pair of proper exercise shoes, most exercises are not expensive to begin with.

As mentioned in the earlier section of this chapter, apart from choosing the type of activity the client will enjoy, other considerations to make will pertain to the fitness goals of the client, the duration of activity, the frequency, and the intensity. Exercises such as walking, jogging, running, dancing and swimming are some of the common aerobic activities most Singaporeans prefer. The following is a short list of the most common forms of aerobic exercise.

7.6.1 *Walking*

Walking is probably the most common form of long-duration aerobic exercise and is most often recommended for beginning exercisers. It is a very low-impact and low-intensity aerobic activity, very easy to perform even up to few hours on end. Brisk or fast walking up the slopes or gentle hills is one way to increase the intensity of exercise.

Here are useful guidelines for administering a walking exercise programme:

- ❖ Maintain a good 'tall' posture throughout.
- ❖ Keep the head upright, shoulders relaxed and eyes looking straight ahead. Be mindful that the shoulders are not rounded or hunched forward.
- ❖ Make sure in every foot strike, the heel should contact the ground first. Roll over the foot and push-off at the ball of the foot. Most people would not have any issue in regards to this.
- ❖ Watch out for awkward walking techniques. For example, the client may be 'flat-footed' and thus over-pronating while walking. This could lead to injury in the course of the walking programme. Refer to a sports medicine specialist or a podiatrist should this happen.
- ❖ Arms generally swing naturally in a coordinated fashion with leg movements. Keep the elbows close to the side of the body during arm swing in forward and backward motion. Elbows are bent around 90 degrees at faster walking speeds.
- ❖ Avoid wide swinging actions that cause the hands to cross the midline of the body.

7.6.2 *Jogging or running*

Running is an all-time favourite aerobic activity with most people. It can be anywhere and anytime, be it on a track, on a treadmill, along the road in housing estates, through the nature reserve treks, etc. Like walking, the investment is low-cost, mostly a pair of shoes, and perhaps some exercise shirts and shorts. The net energy cost for running is higher than walking, hence running is definitely an effective activity for weight maintenance programme.

Because running is a high-impact activity, individuals who are overweight may find activities such as fast walking, swimming or cycling more suitable. For those who prefer exercising with a partner or in a group, there are several running clubs in Singapore that clients can consider joining.

Here are useful guidelines for administering a jogging or running exercise programme:

❖ Start off slowly and gradually work up the pace, distance and running time to meet the desired exercise goals.

❖ For beginners, depending on entry level of fitness, it may be necessary to begin with a walking programme till the client can comfortably complete a distance of more than 5 km without much exertion before alternating walking and running in a session next.

❖ Gradually increase the running time over a few weeks until the client is able to sustain continuous running for at least 20minutes.

❖ Ensure an upright 'tall' posture when running.

❖ Keep the head upright, shoulders relaxed and eyes looking straight ahead. Be mindful that the shoulders are not rounded or hunched forward.

❖ The foot should not be landing out to the side or inward, and there is no need to slam the foot hard onto the ground. The foot should contact the ground lightly with the heel first, roll over and push-off at the ball of the foot.

❖ There is no need to bounce up too high when running. Aim for a smooth, natural forward motion, not up and down motion.

❖ Arms hang relaxed from the shoulders and swing naturally in a coordinated fashion with leg movements. The elbows are bent and the forearms move with the swing between the levels of the chest and hip.

❖ The wrists are relaxed, but not to the point where it caused the hands to loosely hang down from the wrists. Hands are just gently cupped and should not be clenched into fists.

❖ Avoid wide swinging actions that cause the hands to cross the midline of the body.

7.6.3 *Aerobics classes*

Aerobics is also an effective activity for maintenance or training of aerobic fitness. Most of the time, a qualified aerobic instructor is required. People who like the social element of exercise and have a sense of rhythm will enjoy participating in aerobic classes. Classes are affordable, but the client will have to invest in a good pair of aerobic shoes with sufficient padding and ankle support.

There are different basic types of aerobics such as low-impact, high-impact, and step aerobics, as well as modern variations:

❖ Low-impact aerobics moves always maintain one foot on the ground, hence this form of aerobics is good for beginners and those who are heavier in body weight.

❖ High-impact aerobics typically involve a combination of running, hopping and jumping movements and will require both feet to leave the ground momentarily. Although it would be an appropriate vigorous aerobic activity for advanced exercisers, this form of aerobics is not suitable for unconditioned beginners, those with foot injuries and those with special conditions such as pregnancy and overweight issues.

❖ Step aerobics which can be either low-impact or high-impact, or a combination of both, utilize an adjustable raised platform for the aerobic routine moves. The adjustable height of the platform allows clients to work up the exercise intensity as they improve. This form of aerobics has many 'stepping up' and 'stepping down' movements within its routine and may not be suitable for those with knee problems.

❖ Modern variations include incorporating a combination of high-low impact movements, and/or boxing and martial arts moves into the aerobic routines. Such variations are enjoyable and popular among young people.

❖ Aerobics can also be performed in the water, and this form of aerobics is known as water aerobics. Water aerobics are done in waist-high water, thus there is no requirement for anyone to be excellent swimmers. Water aerobics is very low-impact and not strenuous on the knee joints. Such an activity is appropriate for overweight people due to better buoyancy in the water, as well as suitable for clients who are older, pregnant, and those having back or joint problems.

7.6.4 *Dancing*

Dancing is fast gaining popularity among people of all age groups. There are various types of dancing available for those who are interested in participating in this form of exercise. In Singapore, it is quite common to find more middle-aged and older adults participating in somewhat traditional, cultural, social and group-based dancing classes such as folk dance, line dance and ballroom dance. These forms of dancing generally involve routines and recallable steps in their moves and are not too strenuous.

Younger adults may prefer faster moves, jazzy, more exotic and contemporary forms of dancing such as belly dance, hip-hop and modern creative dance. Such forms of dancing tend to involve large, whole body movements over big range of motions across the joints. Workouts are usually of higher-intensity and may require stronger muscular contractions in holding poses.

Dancing classes, including ballet dance class that is supposedly more technical-based, are also readily available for young children and such courses, other than being offered by private dancing studios, are also offered in schools as extra curriculum activities. Fees for dancing classes, usually charged for a fixed number of sessions, may vary, but overall reasonable and affordable. Other costs up-front will be for the purchase of a pair of exercise shoes appropriate for dancing, some exercise tops and stretchable pants. There is a likelihood that people who are new to dancing may feel themselves a little inhibited in the beginning, but will

soon find the fun in dancing classes as their sense of rhythm and
coordination, other than fitness, improves over time.

7.6.5 *Swimming*

Swimming is also another popular activity among Singaporeans. There is
at least one swimming pool in every housing estate across the island.
Swimming generally involves whole body movements in the execution
of swimming strokes. The client can get good aerobic benefits from a
continuous swim of either a long-duration, low-intensity workout or a
short-duration, high-intensity workout.

Because swimming is a non-weight bearing activity, it is suitable for
individuals who are overweight and those with joint or back problems.
However, being a non-weight bearing activity, the contribution to bone
density is minimum, thus it may be necessary to incorporate other
weight-bearing exercises into the training programme in order to meet
client's exercise goals and needs.

Swimming is also seen as a preferred activity by many paraplegic
individuals and people with minor handicap conditions, particularly
those with access to swimming pool and proper supervision. Even for
injured or recovering athletes who are undergoing rehabilitation,
swimming activities and deep water running (i.e. mimick dry-land
running motion) are often prescribed as alternatives to dry-land activities.

For the client who wishes to learn how to swim, there are readily
available lessons conducted by certified swimming instructors at most
swimming pools. Course fees are mostly reasonable. The client will
require a good fitting pair of goggles, and a comfortable swimming suit.
However, most people may take a while to learn the swimming strokes
as swimming generally requires a higher level of skill, involving a
combination of breathing techniques and bodily coordination.

For beginners who have newly learnt one or two swimming strokes, it
may be better to start out the continuous swim at shallower end of the
pool and gradually build up the confidence to manage at the deeper end.

Start the swim at low intensity for up to 10 minutes before building
up towards a higher intensity swim for the next 20-30 minutes. Gradually
work up your time of swim over the period of the training programme.

Some clients may experience cramps halfway through the exercise session. Should this happen, stop swimming and perform some light static stretches over affected joints. If cramps persist, refer the client to a medical specialist.

7.6.6 *Road biking and mountain biking*

Cycling is becoming popular due to the provision of cycling treks in parks and housing estates. Cycling is also a non-weight bearing exercise that is suitable for the overweight and the elderly person, and can be performed either indoor or outdoor.

Weather may be a concern for cycling in the outdoors, hence stationary cycling is seen as convenient and preferred by many. For outdoor cycling, the client needs to purchase a bicycle, which could range from around a hundred dollars to a few thousand dollars depending on the model, function and quality.

Even the most basic bicycle today comes with adjustable handlebar and seat height functions. The height of the seat should be adjusted to a comfortable level where the leg is almost fully extended with a slight knee bent and the foot at the bottom of the down-stroke motion of cycling. If the seat is too low, there will be excessive knee flexion in the cyclic motion and the leg muscles will tire more easily. The seat of the bicycle should be padded with cushions for more comfortable ride. Other than wearing a pair of exercise shoes, it is important to put on a helmet when cycling as well. A light and a back reflector should be attached to the bicycle for cycling in the night.

Cycling accommodate any entry fitness levels. Intensity can be easily monitored with adjustable gear shift function. For example, when pedaling up a slope or hill, change to a higher pedaling cadence (r.p.m.) by shifting the gears to reduce the amount of exerting force while pedaling upwards. The client can also choose a pedaling speed that suits his or her fitness level and comfort.

Always begin each cycling session slowly at a low level of resistance for up to 10 minutes. Progressively increase in the intensity and duration of exercise over time. Ensure the tires are properly inflated, and most importantly, avoid cycling around vehicles or cycling in areas of heavy traffic or pollution.

7.6.7 *Rollerblading or in-line skating*

Rollerblading is also known as in-line skating, and is a modern day variation of ice skating and traditional roller skates. Another similar aerobic leisure activity rising in participation rate is ice-skating. The ice-skating rings available in Singapore can accommodate up to one hundred people or more in a single session, although the speed of skating is vastly limited in a crowded space.

Rollerblading as an aerobic exercise is gaining popularity among the young people in Singapore and you can find many enthusiasts, and even children, skating away skilfully in the parks and along the beach paths. Although the traffic system is effective in Singapore, the heavy and fast moving traffic makes it unsafe and inappropriate for skaters to take this form of exercise to the streets.

Most people may find it challenging to balance on the skate and may take some time to learn skating with coordination and skill. For beginners, it is recommended for lessons to be conducted in a large enclosed space and controlled environment to achieve some degree of skill and confidence. Most classes provide the specialized equipment such as the skates, helmet and protective gears packed into the course fees, or it is also possible to rent such equipment cheaply at many locations in parks and beach areas. Otherwise, for clients who like to take up this form of exercise long-term, buying a pair of in-line skates and a fitting helmet and protective gears is definitely a good investment for health and wellness.

7.6.8 *Rope skipping*

Rope skipping is a very effective and high-impact aerobic activity, but may not be suitable for some people, particularly those who more senior, those who are overweight and those who have lower limb joint issues. Rope skipping provides a whole body workout involving largely the lower body, as well as arms and grip work. Many serious exercisers and athletes incorporate this mode of exercise into their training routines for more effective results, or as a variation to other forms of aerobic workouts.

Successful skipping will require certain level of skill and coordination. Simple single- and double-legged jumps are easier to perform than variations such as single leg alternating, forward motions, backward motions, sideways motions, double-turns, alternate crisscross and crossovers. Make sure the client has a good pair of exercise shoes with sufficient cushioning. The skipping rope is not expensive to buy, and the rope materials range from plastic to heavy nylon types.

Choosing a heavier rope will result in a more intense workout. For those who have already attained a good level of overall physical fitness but new to skipping, they can embark slowly in the beginning and gradually build up the exercise intensity, duration of continuous skipping, as well as increase the variation or styles of skipping for added enjoyment.

7.6.9 *Stair climbing*

Who would have thought that stair-climbing could be a good aerobic exercise for Singaporeans? The benefits derived from regular stair-climbing exercise are widely documented. This form of exercise has been shown to be effective in improving cardiovascular fitness, reducing cholesterol levels, decreasing body fat, and particularly, increasing the strength of the lower limbs. It has been shown that stair-climbing activity elicits oxygen and heart rate responses that meet the minimum intensity requirements set by ASCM for cardiorespiratory and health gains.

The value of stair-climbing as an exercise mode for the masses is even more relevant to countries like Singapore, a land-scarce island where more than 80% of its population live in government-built high-rise flats. It is a low-cost option and provides convenience to all who are able to access public stairs. The intensity of exercise can vary with the pace of climbing and beginners can choose to begin slowly for shorter duration of exercise, and even take intermittent short period of rest after every few levels of ascend.

7.6.10 *Aerobic exercise in the form of organised sports*

There are other effective aerobic activities in the form of organized sports such as badminton, soccer, basketball, rollerblade hockey and tennis being some of the more common ones. All of these activities provide general cardiovascular benefits although training programmes can be designed in a way to build up specific physical capacities. However, there are activities such as golf, billiard and bowling that do not provide as much cardiovascular benefits.

Most of the population who participate in these activities would enjoy more of the social elements, have fun in the company of friends and family while at the same time develop some levels of fitness. For the client who is also an athlete, he or she may prefer training programmes that are planned with the aim of developing both skill and specific components of fitness through practices of skills and techniques.

Regardless of the exercise motives and goals, minimally to achieve some aerobic benefits, the exercise should permit sustained active or repetitive movements using large muscle groups for at least 30 minutes. This way, intensity of exercise may still be meeting the minimum guideline of at least 60% of maximum heart rate. It may be difficult to continue participating in the same organized sports activity at least 3 days a week, hence throwing a session of such an activity into a weekly programme provides variation and helps prevent boredom.

For additional benefit for clients with young children, the trainer can even make this unique session per week a family activity. Apart from gaining health benefits for young children, game activities played together can help to form the base for family bonding as early as possible.

7.6.11 *Circuit training*

Although circuit training is known as the simplest and most common method used to develop general strength capacity for sports performance, it can also be used for most of the population, including overweight individuals and older adults, to develop non-specific aerobic capacity by combining elements of weight and endurance training. Even for athletes, such training method will apply well to aerobic-dominant sports.

With circuit training method, different muscle groups can be worked alternately from station to station. Besides utilising available weight training machines in the gym, a wide variety of body weight exercises and exercises using devices such as surgical tubing, medicine balls, light implements, dumbbells can also be used in a circuit training routine. Adding variety keeps the client interested and, at the same time, constantly challenges the client's learning aptitude and skill.

A circuit may be of short (6 to 9 exercises) to long (12 to 15 exercises) duration and may be repeated several times depending on the number of exercises involved. Trainers must consider the client's work tolerance and fitness level when planning for the number of circuits, the number of repetitions per station, and the load/resistance used. Total workload in a workout session should not be so high as to cause pain or high discomfort.

The following guidelines apply to training for circuit training:

- ❖ Alternate muscle groups in exercises planned for the circuit session. For example, alternating exercises targeting shoulder (i.e. deltoid muscle) to hip (thigh adductors/abductors) to arm (triceps muscle) to calf (gastrocnemius muscle), and so on.
- ❖ Set up a number of stations that aim to work the entire body.
- ❖ Use light weights or loads that the client can lift for 15 to 25 repetitions without causing great fatigue.
- ❖ Each exercise can be performed continuously for a specified time interval, e.g. 1 minute at each station, or the exercise can be performed from 1 to 3 sets of a certain number of repetitions. After a set of repetitions at an exercise station, the client may move on to another station and complete the whole cycle of other stations before coming back to do another set.
- ❖ Some circuit training routines include short periods of 10 minutes treadmill work, skipping or cycling in between stations to add variety. The focus here is not entirely for strength gains, but varying routines for aerobic workout. This type of routine seems to be suitable for keeping up motivation of elderly clients.

❖ If the intention is to split a session into two components: weights and aerobic workout, it will be better to do weights training section first before the aerobic section.

7.7 Cardiovascular Machines and Equipment

In almost every gym today, it is common to find machines that are specifically designed for cardiovascular work, and the most common types are treadmills, stationary bicycles, stair climbers, rowing machines and elliptical trainers. Most of these machines come with electronic functions making it convenient to adjust speed and resistance of exercise. Having cardiovascular machines indoor also means clients can enjoy exercising regardless of weather, and often in the comfort of conducive, air-conditioned environment.

7.7.1 *Treadmills*

Treadmills are used for stationary walking or running and similarly effective in expending calories. Most of the treadmills come in motorized models while there are some self-powered forms. Clients can easily program the treadmill to go fast or slow, flat or incline using the electronic monitoring device situated in front of the treadmill.

Most treadmills have pre-programmed routines (e.g. fat loss, fartlek, interval training, hills) built into its electronic monitoring system for varied workouts. All treadmills, no matter how basic, will come with a handrail and at least one emergency stop button that once pressed will trigger an emergency stop in the event of losing balance, unstable walking or running movements or nearly slipping off.

Here are safety guidelines that the client must be made aware of before performing any treadmill exercise:

❖ To begin exercising on the treadmill, start by straddling the sides of the treadmill holding the handrail with two hands at a comfortable distance apart. Do not start by standing on top of the belt.

❖ Always start the belt of the treadmill moving at a low speed. When the belt has started moving, get used to the belt movement by having one foot moving with the belt several times before stepping on with the other foot.

❖ In the beginning stages, the client may still have the hands on the handrail while walking or jogging on the belt. To slowly build a client's confidence to let go of the handrail, it may take a while or over few sessions. The trainer needs to be patient in applying the following method to help the client in this aspect:
  o start by holding the handrail with the fingers gently;
  o moving on to one hand hold while swinging the other arm naturally at the side;
  o proceed to holding the rail with only the fingers of one hand;
  o finally releasing the handrail with both arms swinging by the side of the body.

❖ Walk or jog as naturally as possible and not try to lean forward.

❖ Always stay in the center of the belt.

❖ Eyes should be looking forward at all times.

❖ Avoid turning to the side while talking to someone. If necessary to have a conversation, it will be best to hold on to the handrails for that moment.

❖ In the event of losing balance, unstable walking or running movements or nearly slipping off, hit the emergency stop button. The belt will slow down drastically but keep walking until the belt comes to a complete stop.

7.7.2 *Stationary bicycles*

Stationary cycling simulates real cycling except that the exerciser does not require the skill and balance needed for outdoor cycling. Furthermore, because of its non-weight bearing and non-impact activity nature, it is one of the most preferred machines used by overweight individuals and older adults, as well as those who lower limb injuries or joint problems.

Cycling cadence and resistance can be easily changed as most of the bicycle ergometers use a flywheel, strap or air resistance systems to add or substract loads. There are two basic types of bicycle ergometers: the classic upright type and the recumbent or reclining type. Most bicycle ergometers come with softer or cushioned seats, but it may still feel uncomfortable for the buttocks when cycling for long duration.

The classic upright model also comes with an adjustable handlebar. There is a variation to the upright model which comes with arm levers that allow 'push and pull' movements to provide accompanying workout to the upper body. The height of the seat can be adjusted to a comfortable level where the leg is almost fully extended with a slight knee bent. This ensures a good posture for cycling whereby the thigh alignment is somewhat parallel to the floor and the knee is not above the hips when the pedal is moved to its upmost stroke position.

Good posture also means that the back and shoulders are not hunched and rounded even though the torso should be tilted slightly forward. The handlebar in front allows a comfortable hold at about shoulder width apart although the height and position of the handlebar is a matter of individual choice in terms of comfort and preference.

For example, a cyclist may prefer to adopt a racing body position by placing the forearm on the sides of the handlebar. An older exerciser may prefer a more upright posture and a higher handlebar position for better comfort. In any case, the elbows should not be tensed or 'locked', but remain relaxed with a slight bent.

The recumbent bicycle requires the exerciser to sit back into a seat with the upper body supported by a backrest. The pedals are in front and situated slightly below the level of the seat. Likewise, the seat can be adjusted forward or backward to allow for slight knee bent at leg extension. The recumbent bicycle usually comes with handlebars on both sides of the seat. This allows the exerciser to have a relaxed grip whilst cycling yet maintained a 'tall' back posture against the backrest. Alternatively, there is also a handlebar situated in front of the chest position about slightly less than an arm length distance away.

7.7.3 *Stair climbers*

There are many models of stair climbers in the market. The basic, cheaper models work on simple hydraulic systems that permit a much shallower stepping depth which may not adequate engage the working muscles, predominantly the gluteal, hamstring and quadriceps muscles. Stair climbers that come with independently moving pedals will allow a more realistic simulation of actual stair climbing actions and thus enable a more effective workout as compared to pedal mechanics that automatically brings one pedal up while the other goes down.

The stair climber provides a low-impact exercise alternative to actual stair climbing and is suitable for almost all entry levels of fitness. However, this activity may not be ideal for individuals with knee problems. If this exercise produces pain at the joint and high levels of discomfort, stop immediately. The trainer should then recommend a more appropriate activity for the client.

Stair climbers come with handrails by on both sides of the machine allowing exercisers to hold on lightly for support and balance. However, be mindful not to lean on the handrail to seek more support for body weight. This will decrease the effectiveness of the exercise considerably. Those with back problems should not lean over excessively as this will cause more strain on the lower back. Maintain an upright "tall" posture throughout the exercise. Avoid side-to-side hip movements, which is likely to occur with a stepping depth over and beyond what the individual can manage.

Most stair climbers allow a stepping depth of between 10 to 20 centimeters. It is therefore good to choose a stair climber that allows control of stepping depth. While stepping, keep the toes forward and the feet parallel to the pedals. Keep the whole foot in contact with the pedal while stepping and avoid 'pressing down' with the balls of the feet as this may cause unnecessary strain to the ankles. The pedals should not be moved all the down to the floor or all the way up to the extreme end of the range of movement.

Of course, choosing a stair climber that is stable without any wobble is also important, particularly for overweight exercisers or individuals with big body frames and musculature. For beginners, go for a

comfortable stepping speed that will not cause poor posture and
excessive side-to-side movements. As the client improves, gradually
work up the stepping speed and duration of exercise.

7.7.4 *Rowing machines*

The rowing exercise performed on a rowing machine with a moving seat
on a track closely simulates the actual movement of rowing a boat. This
activity actually provides a great all-round whole body aerobic workout
involving many muscles of the upper and lower body.

Indoor rowing is a non-impact and non weight-bearing activity and
therefore is quite a good alternative for those who have orthopaedic
problems and overweight individuals. However, it is recommended that
they first attain a foundational level of fitness before embarking on this
form of exercise. Rowing may not be the sole exercise for the training of
aerobic fitness, but it can definitely be incorporated as a component of
the overall aerobic training programme to add variety.

The client needs to understand the movements involved in this
rowing exercise. The rowing motion itself requires a great deal of
coordination and most beginners may find it hard or make mistakes that
cause strain on the body parts, particularly the lower back.

It is important to keep the torso straight and the lower back arched by
holding the core muscles tight. For this exercise, the lower back should
not be rounded. Keeping the torso straight will prevent the shoulders
from hunching. The forward and backward leaning movements of the
torso natural come from the hips as a result of the well-executed rowing
motions. The trainer must constantly remind the client to maintain a good
posture right from the start and throughout the full rowing motion.

The number of strokes (cadence) is usually kept approximately 20 to
30 rows per minute. It is more important to perform at a manageable
cadence with proper technique than to row fast with poor technique. The
latter when done excessively without proper technique and control can
cause unnecessary strain to body parts and may lead to injury. Like other
exercise, start at a slower cadence and gradually work up the pace.

Pay attention to the following details when performing the full
rowing motion:

❖ Begin by sitting on the movable seat of the rowing machine. Secure the feet to the foot straps of the foot pedals that are placed at a fixed positioned along the track of the rowing machine.

❖ Lean the body slightly forward, knees are brought close to the chest, and hands holding on to the handle. The arms are extended straight in front while holding the handle, and keeping the hands slightly below the level of the shoulders.

❖ Keep the head upright with the eyes looking forward and the back straightened upright.

❖ Push the foot pedals with the legs forcefully using the muscles of the gluteals, hips and quadriceps. At this driving point, the seat moves backward along the track while the hands are holding the handle with arms outstretched, the torso leans back slightly from the hips.

❖ Towards the end of the push when the hips and knees are extended, the elbows flex while pulling the handle towards the abdomen at just below the level of the rib cage.

❖ The elbows should stay close to the body while flexing (i.e. elbows pointing more towards the back while pulling) and not be abducted excessively from the body (i.e. elbows pointing too laterally to the side while pulling).

❖ The hands must not begin the pull until the hips and knees are extended. This is to prevent the arm muscles from fatiguing too early.

❖ All the while throughout this motion from the start to the end of the push, the back is kept straight with a slight backward lean.

❖ Recovering back to the starting point begins with the arms extending forward, and the torso slightly leaning forward while bringing the handle to pass the point of the knees. In the course of recovering, the forward lean will still maintain the torso in a vertical position.

❖ Do not lean forward excessively such that torso passes over the vertical line at this point. It is important that the back remains straightened and abdomen muscles tightened.

❖ The arms stretching forward is an intentional effort to keep the tension of the handle pulling on the arms forward. As the handle passes the point of the knees, the hips and knees flex and the seat moves forward along the track towards the front of the machine.

❖ Towards the end of the recovery, the seat comes close to the front of the machine, the torso leans pass the vertical line and the knees close to the chest.

❖ The arms extends straight in front while holding the handle. This is the starting position once again, and the next stroke is ready to begin.

❖ Remember to exhale while pushing the foot pedals and pulling the handle, and inhale while recovering to the starting position.

7.7.5 *Elliptical cross trainers*

Exercising on an elliptical cross trainer is a popular choice for many because it provides an interesting, low-impact aerobic workout. The feet contact the pedals that move in an elliptical path continuously and in a somewhat similar motion to running except without the impact of actual running on the ground or treadmill.

The machine may come with electronic selection functions to choose either forward or reversed leg motions. Pedalling in reverse motions allows conditioning of a different set of muscles. Resistance and intensity of exercise can also be set by the exerciser based on individual preferences.

Although an elliptical cross trainer is primarily designed to provide aerobic workouts that involve more of the lower body, there are elliptical trainers that come with arm levers that allow 'push and pull' movements to provide accompanying workout to the upper body. Otherwise, all elliptical cross trainers should come with handrails for light support and balance. Do not lean on the handrail to seek more support for body weight as this will compromise the effectiveness of the exercise considerably.

Always adopt a "tall" upright posture. Keep the head up and eyes looking forward throughout the duration of the exercise. Make sure the knees do not cross forward over the toes while pedalling in elliptical movements. This may happen if the client leans forward excessively or rely more on the handrail for supporting the body weight. Keep the torso balance and directly above the hips while pedalling.

Older or simpler models may come with fixed pedals and restricted motion paths. Newer or improved models allow adjustment to be made to the pedal positions (i.e. straight or inclined), speed of pedalling (cadence), and the range of motion paths (i.e. change in stride length). When the pedals are inclined, the movements simulate stair climbing. Otherwise, without much pedal inclination, depending on the cadence, movements will simulate either walking or running motions. Some machines have electronic selection functions that come with preset exercise programmes for exercisers to choose their preferred exercise settings.

7.8 Monitoring Intensity of Cardiovascular Conditioning

To ensure and account for optimal benefits from the participation of aerobic workouts, there is a need to more objectively monitor the exercise intensity of the client.

7.8.1 *Measuring the heart rate (HR)*

The simplest and accurate way to monitor exercise intensity is by monitoring the heart rate or pulse. HR increases linearly with work intensity. Generally, the higher the intensity of the exercise, the higher the heart rate is expected, and in reverse, the lower the intensity of the exercise, the lower the heart rate is expected.

HR is commonly used to determine a client's target heart rate or training zone for aerobic workouts. Availability of HR telemetric systems makes it easy to monitor HR during exercise, and HR values can also be stored and retrieved which enables immediate feedback during exercise and post exercise. HR can be checked against other physiological or subjective markers of intensity.

There are 2 preferred ways to measure and monitor the client's heart rate:

7.8.1.1 *Taking the pulse*

Feel the pulse at the radial artery site of the wrist. Use the index and middle fingers to palpate the pulse. Count and measure the number of pulse beats for at least 10 seconds. Convert to beats per minute (bpm) by multiplying the value by 6. This is preferred to the common carotid artery site at the neck.

Place the fingers on the side of the windpipe just below the jaw to palpate the pulse. Pressing hard on the neck is uncomfortable and pressure on the vagus nerve situated in the same region nearby may send signals to slow the heart rate, giving a false lower pulse reading.

As soon as the exercise stops and the client needs to feel and count the heart rate, do bear in mind that the heart rate will start to recover and slow down especially after an exercise where the intensity has been high. If the client takes too long to measure the heart rate, the value may not be as accurate. Hence, measuring the pulse counts for at least 10 seconds will provide a more accurate value than if the pulse count is measured over a period of 30 seconds or a minute.

7.8.1.2 *Using a heart rate monitor*

These are simple digital devices that mostly come in form of wrist watches with a sensor strapped across the chest that can be worn by the client during exercise. In recent years the prices of these devices have become much more affordable for the individual and can be very handy for personal trainers to own at least a set.

There are also many cardiovascular machines that already come with touch sensitive pads on the handlebars that allow registering of the electrical signals of the heart beat. Whenever the client requires immediately feedback of exercise heart rate, grab onto the handlebars firmly, but not too tightly, and the exercise heart rate value will appear very shortly. It is advisable that before working out on a cardiovascular machine, clean the pads of the handlebars by wiping with an exercise towel to ensure hygiene.

7.8.2 *Resting heart rate (RHR)*

Most people have RHR of between 60 to 80 beats per minute. On average, females tend to have a higher RHR than males by up to 10 beats. For RHR, it will be better to count the pulse over 30 seconds and then multiply the value by 2. This heart rate reflects the lowest end of the range of one's heart rate. Hence ideally, it should be measured immediately after the client wakes up and before getting out of bed.

An average of several days' readings should be calculated for a more reliable record. This value is useful to monitor current state of recovery or fitness. For instance, an elevated morning RHR approximately 20 to 40% above the normal range consistently could indicate that the body has not fully recovered from previous exercise sessions.

When the client has participated in an exercise programme regularly over a period of time, as the heart gets fitter, it takes less beats to pump the same amount of blood as it did before, the RHR also gets lower.

7.8.3 *Maximum heart rate (HRmax)*

A person's maximum heart rate is the theoretical number of beats per minute that the heart is capable of producing. The HRmax can be estimated by subtracting one's age from 220. For example, a 35 year old client has a HRmax of 185 (220 – 35).

The above formula, while useful and simple to compute, does not take into consideration the cardiovascular fitness level of clients. According to ACSM guidelines, this formula tends to either overestimate (age 20-40) or underestimate (age >40) by up to 10 to 12 bpm.

7.8.4 *Establish training HR range*

Establishing individual client training zones will assist the trainer in the planning of the aerobic workout sessions. This will provide a guide from training too hard or too easy and at the same time help the client to adhere to reasonable training goals. It also provides the client safe targets to aim for even when training hard.

7.8.4.1   *Percent of maximum heart rate method*

Below is an example of determining a range of training heart rates based on a percentage of the HRmax. The training target zone accommodates an appropriate training intensity range of between 0.6 (220-Age) to 0.9 (220-Age).

Table 7.7. Determining a range of training heart rates based on a percentage of the HRmax.

Calculating Lower Limit Heart Rate (e.g. a 35 year old person with resting heart rate of 68 bpm)	
Maximal heart rate	185 bpm
x 60%	x .6
Equals lower limit heart rate	*111 bpm*
Calculating Upper Limit Heart Rate	
Maximal heart rate	185 bpm
x 90%	x .9
Equals upper limit heart rate	*166 bpm*

7.8.4.2   *Calculating heart rate reserve (HHR)*

A more sensitive training intensity for aerobic conditioning is the Karvonen Formula. The desired training percentage for this formula is 50-85%.

The mathematical formula is given as:

$$HHR = HRmax - HRrest$$

The training HHR zone is calculated as:

[Lower limit percent HRR minus Upper limit percent HHR] + HRrest,
or simply,
%(HRmax – HRrest) + HRrest.

Below is an example of determining the training zone using the Karvonen formula.

Table 7.8. Determining the training zone using the Karvonen formula.

Calculating Heart Rate Reserve	
(e.g. a 35 year old person with resting heart rate of 68 bpm)	
Maximal heart rate	185 bpm
Minus resting heart rate	- 68 bpm
Equals heart rate reserve (HRR)	*117 bpm*
Calculating Lower Limit Heart Rate	
HRR	117 bpm
x 50%	x .5
Equals	58 bpm
Plus resting heart rate	+68 bpm
Equals lower limit heart rate	*126 bpm*
Calculating Upper Limit Heart Rate	
HRR	117 bpm
x 85%	x .85
Equals	100 bpm
Plus resting heart rate	+68 bpm
Equals upper limit heart rate	*168 bpm*

7.8.5 *Ratings of perceived exertion (RPE)*

The rating of perceived exertion (RPE) is not a substitute for heart rate (HR). RPE may not always or consistently translate to the same intensity for different modes of exercise.

Table 7.9. An example adapted from the
original Borg RPE scale.

Rating	Description
6 7	Very, very light
8 9	Very light
10 11	Fairly light
12 13	Somewhat hard
14 15	Hard
16 17	Very hard
18 19	Very, very hard
20	Maximal

7.8.6 *Signs or symptoms of exertion using Talk Test*

Use the talk test to estimate exercise intensity. It is not about whether the talk test is a "good" or "bad" thing, but it is about what is appropriate for the client.

A client should be able to hold a short conversation without being too breathless while exercising. If talking becomes increasingly difficulty, the exercise intensity is probably too hard.

Personal trainers should teach beginners this useful tip as it 'educates' and empowers the client to take responsibility for listening to his or her body whilst exercising.

Table 7.10. Common safety checks for signs/symptoms whilst client is exercising.

Signs or symptoms from client:	Trainer's decision:
The client is maintaining a "comfortable uncomfortable" sense of feeling whilst exercising.	The client can continue into the next activity.
The client is breathing comfortably throughout given duration of activity.	The client can continue into the next activity.
The client has difficult stringing few words of conversation whilst exercising.	Slow down as most probably has exceeded the anaerobic threshold. Continue to monitor using talk test.
The client expresses a sense of uncomfortable feeling and fatigue in muscles.	Slow down. If muscles are hurting or in pain, stop the activity and find out why. If there is an injury, seek necessary treatment.
The client expresses a need to "really wanting to stop."	Slow down and continue to monitor for some more minutes. If the client still expresses a strong desire to stop, then proceed to other low intensity activity such as slow walk and stretching.

7.9 Action Strategies

Start to plan, and plan to start! It is important to be able to communicate accurately the benefits of having adequate cardiovascular fitness, or aerobic fitness, in daily life across to your client. Aim for understanding of such lifestyle issues, not just knowledge of fitness per se. Make the participation in physical activities and exercises as regular and enjoyable as possible. Adapt to client's needs, interests and lifestyle requirements instead of a 'one size fits all' prescription.

7.10 In the News

Highlight debilitating consequences of poor cardiovascular health. Include incidences of recent sudden cardiac deaths. Highlight advantages of good cardiovascular fitness or health in average men, women, elderly and children. Feature recent examples when educating the client on the importance of maintaining good cardiovascular health.

7.11 Summary and Key Points

Incorporating activities into daily routines is not that difficult. Issues of needs and concerns can be catered for. For the fitness professionals, it' not an issue of 'right' or 'wrong' to do little or lots of activities, rather, it's an issue of appropriateness and encouraging more and more people to be active effectively.

7.12 Recommended Readings and Website Resource

(1) American College of Sports Medicine (1998). Position stand on the recommended quantity and quality of exercise for developing and maintaining cardiovascular and muscular fitness, and flexibility in healthy adults. *Med Sci Sports Exerc*, 30, pp. 975–991.

(2) Chia, M., Leong, L.L. and Quek, J.J. (2004). *Healthy, Well and Wise: Take PRIDE for a Life of Wellness.* National Institute of Education, Singapore. Order details: Office of Graduate Programmes and Professional Learning.

(3) Heyward, V.H. (2002). *Advanced Fitness Assessment and Exercise Prescription.* 4th Ed. Human Kinetics, USA.

(4) Developed by a team of sport specialists from the National Institute of Education, SSSS is a scientific and holistic approach to understanding and practising the principles of science for conditioning for health and fitness. SSSS will help clients get the most out of their sporting pursuits, training, practice or competition: www.sportsuccess.nie.edu.sg

(5) http://www.mayoclinic.com is an award-winning consumer Web site that offers health information, self-improvement and disease management tools. This website contains relevant health and fitness related resources such as healthy living articles, videos and slide shows that fitness professionals will find useful.

Chapter 8

Designing the Nutritional Programme

A person's health and wellness is largely affected by what he eats and drinks. The role of good nutrition for optimal health cannot be underestimated. As a personal trainer, you are one of those your client is likely to seek nutritional advice from. Thus, you are also the most likely person who can teach and impart sound nutritional knowledge, thereby influencing your client to make wise and good decisions for life-long healthy eating.

After completing this chapter, you will be able to:

- ❖ Understand and apply sound knowledge of nutrition.
- ❖ Provide appropriate nutritional advice to clients.
- ❖ Recommend healthy eating strategies and modify recipes and diets for different needs.
- ❖ Understand effective weight management based on scientific principles.
- ❖ Understand eating behaviours and eating disorders.

8.1 Introduction

Most individuals are aware that what they eat and drink has an impact on their well-being and health. However, many still find it difficult to deliberately plan and eat healthily, predominantly due to hectic lifestyles and lack of knowledge. The abundance and convenience of cheaper food options available at hawker centres and food courts does not help. On the other side of the spectrum are a small though growing number of individuals who will pay attention to special diets or invest in expensive supplements to achieve a higher level of wellness or attain certain desired physical performance or physical changes.

Clients are constantly asking questions that seek to address concerns on 'weighty' issues, pursuing the 'perfect' body, improving appearance, and even what they can eat to help them work, study, or sleep better. Today, there are also individuals who are particularly interested in finding out ways to eat their way out of sickness and aging. Regardless, the lack of consistency in the nutrition business and media reports make it harder to convey sound and realistic messages to clients in regards to what would be good for them – which is a combination of keeping physically active and happy, and eating wisely.

Personal trainers who understand sound concepts of healthy nutrition are in a good position to help clear clients' doubts and confusions and provide the right nutrition and health guidance. In this way, they are also in the position to boost clients' confidence for life-long healthy eating habits.

8.2 Professional Role of the Personal Trainer in Nutrition

The professional role of the trainer in working with the client in a nutritional programme ought to be a credible and sensible one – one that is able to convey messages that become a part of the client's overall health and wellness picture. He or she should be able to advise and guide the client to take on and make sound nutritional decisions for life.

8.3 What is a Healthy Diet?

A healthy well-balanced diet in relation to health, exercise and energy balance is one that provides energy and nutrients to meet the needs of the body for its daily activities, promotes good health and optimises exercise performance. Although there may be special groups of individuals (i.e. women athletes, vegetarians) who require more specialized diets, for most of the population, eating a wide variety of foods from each of the food groups in the Healthy Diet Pyramid is a good guide.

The Healthy Diet Pyramid includes the recommended servings and portions used in Singapore. The figure below shows the proportion of foods from the different food groups that make up a healthy diet.

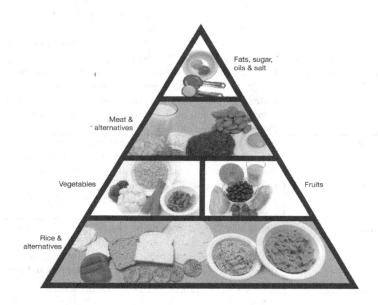

Fig. 8.1. Recommended Healthy Diet Pyramid.

To determine if the client is meeting the Healthy Diet Pyramid recommendations, the trainer can ask the client to keep a 24-hour to 72-hour record of his or her own diet by tallying the number of portions consumed during each meal. Portions could be recorded with sufficient details such as 'drink half a cup of milk before bedtime', 'ate 2 bananas and half a blueberry muffin and drank a cup of milo for breakfast'.

Below are some interpretations of serving size according to the Healthy Diet Pyramid recommendations. In this chapter, we particularly choose to highlight more on common Asian foods in our examples as these foods are not extensively mentioned or discussed in most publications. Asian foods are also becoming popular around the world. The same principles can definitely be applied to other food types as well.

Table 8.1. Interpretations of serving size according to the Healthy Diet Pyramid recommendations.

Rice and Alternatives	Eat 5-7 servings (or more) daily. These foods provide carbohydrates for energy. Go for wholegrain products such as wholemeal bread and unpolished or brown rice more often. 1 serving in Asian food proportion could be equivalent to 2 slices of chappati, ½ rice bowl of rice or noodles, or 1 rice bowl of porridge.
Fats, Oil, Sugar and Salt	Choose small amounts of unsaturated fats (e.g. margarine, or corn, soybean, canola or olive oils) instead of saturated fats (e.g. butter, lard, blended vegetable or palm oils). Use sugars and salt sparingly to enhance the taste of food.
Meat and Alternatives	Eat 2-3 servings daily. 1 serving is equivalent to 80-90g of cooked meat, poultry or fish (or about one palm-size), 4-5 medium-sized prawns, 2-3 small squares of tofu, 2-3 eggs, ¾ cup of legumes (e.g. beans, dhal), 2-3 cups of milk, 1 small tub of yoghurt or 2 slices of cheese.
Vegetables	Eat at least 2-3 servings daily. Go for variations of fresh or cooked green- or orange-coloured vegetables (e.g. chye sim, spinach, broccoli, carrot, and tomato) instead of frozen vegetables. 1 serving is equivalent to ¾-1 cup of cooked vegetables or 150-200g raw vegetables.
Fruits	Eat at least 2-3 servings daily. An example of 1 serving equivalent is 1 apple, orange or pear, 1 medium-sized banana or 1 slice papaya or melon.

8.4 Estimated Energy Expenditure of Various Sports and Physical Activities

Energy found in food and used for physical activity is measured in kilocalories (kcal) or kilojoules (kJ). A person's energy requirements vary with his/her height, weight, gender, age, metabolic rate (the way the body uses up energy), and physical activity.

Table 8.2. The three nutrients that contribute to estimated energy.

Nutrient	Energy (kcal) per gram
Carbohydrate	4
Protein	4
Fat	9

8.4.1 *Carbohydrates*

Carbohydrates are readily available source of energy for muscle contraction during most types of exercise. During digestion, carbohydrates are broken down into glucose.

Table 8.3. A guide to the amounts of carbohydrate that can be consumed according to the various levels of exercise.

Exercise Intensity	Duration	Carbohydrate (g/kg/day)
Light	< 1 hr	4.0 – 4.5
Light/Moderate	1 hr	4.5 – 5.0
Moderate	1 – 2 hr	5.5 – 6.5
Moderate/Heavy	2 – 4 hr	6.5 – 7.5
Heavy	4 – 5 hr	7.5 – 8.5

Table 8.4. Carbohydrate foods in 3 categories.

Nutritious Carbohydrates	Foods providing valuable sources of other nutrients (vitamins, minerals and fibre) are placed in this first and most important group. Choose these foods at each main meal. A lack of these healthier nutritious carbohydrates from the main diet may result in vitamin and mineral deficiencies. Nutritious carbohydrates include wholemeal and multi-grain breads, brown or unpolished rice, pasta, high fibre crackers, high fibre and fortified cereals, fresh fruit, low fat/skimmed milk and yoghurt, starchy vegetables such as potato, sweet potato, corn, and dried beans and lentils.
Refined Carbohydrates	Foods that provide carbohydrate in the form of sugars. These foods include sugar (white, brown and raw), jam and marmalade, honey, sweets, sports drinks, soft drinks, syrups and cordials, popsicles, jelly and sweet Asian-based dessert soups. Do not consume them regularly at meals or as snacks. Clients may have them in moderation from time to time.
High-Fat Carbohydrates	Many of the local Asian favourites (e.g. char kway teow, fried carrot cake, roti prata) are found in this group. Other carbohydrate foods high in fat include cakes and pastries, deep-fried snacks (curry puff, potato chips, french fries), chocolates, ice cream, and some foods made with coconut (e.g. nasi lemak, buboh cha cha). While there is no need to avoid these foods, it is best not to take them regularly at meals or as snacks. Clients may have them as treats and on special occasions. The additional energy from fat can cause unwanted fat tissue gains.

Glucose, the primary fuel for normal body functions and exercising muscles must be maintained within a narrow range in the blood. The more a person exercises, the greater the amount of glucose needed.

Glucose that is not needed for the moment is stored as glycogen in the muscles and the liver. When the need for glucose arises, glycogen stores are broken down and released into the bloodstream. Adequate glycogen stores are essential for working muscles during training. Clients who fail to consume adequate amounts daily while training may have decreased endurance and poorer performance.

During long periods of not eating (i.e. during sleep), the body breaks down some glycogen into glucose to maintain normal blood glucose levels. Skipping meals, especially breakfast, can result in low blood glucose levels if glycogen stores are low. Symptoms of low blood glucose include irritability, lack of ability to focus, headache, muscular weakness, or even fainting. The choice of carbohydrate foods can also affect exercise performance and health.

Here are some ways the client can reduce high-fat carbohydrates when eating out:

❖ Choose soup or dry noodles more frequently than fried noodles.
❖ Ask for steamed rice rather than other types of cooked rice such as briyani, fried or coconut rice.
❖ Ask for less curry-based gravy or soya-based sauces when having rice with dishes, or avoid adding additional salt or soya sauces to dishes served totally.

To meet the body's daily carbohydrate requirements, it is important to know how much carbohydrate foods one needs to actually consume. Use Table 8.5 which comprises of some popular local Singapore foods to practice working out the estimated carbohydrate portions of these foods using this simple system of calculation:

❖ Each portion contains 30g of carbohydrate. For example, 2 slices of bread will add up to approximately 30g which is 1 portion.

Here are additional pointers to compare the Carbohydrate Portions with the Healthy Diet Pyramid recommendation:

❖ For bread, rice, noodles and cereals, 1 Carbohydrate Portion = 1 serving from the Rice and Alternatives group.

❖ For smaller cut fruits, 1 Carbohydrate Portion = 2 servings from the Fruit group.

Table 8.5. Estimated carbohydrate portions of some popular local Singapore foods.

Common Food	Amount	Energy (kcal)	Carbohydrate (g)	Fat (g)	Protein (g)
Braised Duck Rice	1 plate	706	86	30	24
Carrot Cake, Fried with Egg	1 plate	466	51	24	11
Char Kway Teow	1 plate	742	76	39	23
Chicken Rice	1 plate	618	76	23	26
Fishball Mee Soup	1 bowl	329	58	2	18
Fish Porridge	1 bowl	258	40	3	17
Fried Hokkien Mee	1 plate	613	65	30	22
Fried Rice	1 plate	511	66	20	16
Laksa Lemak	1 bowl	587	58	32	17
Mee Siam	1 plate	520	82	15	15
Nasi Lemak	1 packet	279	29	13	12
Roti Prata	1 small	122	19	4	3
Popular Snacks	Amount	Energy (kcal)	Carbohydrate (g)	Fat (g)	Protein (g)
Curry Puff, Chicken	1 piece	246	20	16	5
Pau, Char Siew	1 portion	206	25	8	7
Spring Roll	1 piece	127	8	10	2
Sushi, Assorted	1 piece	30-65	6-10	0-1	1-3
Cake, Pandan Chiffon	1 slice	97	6	7	3
Kuih Lapis, Steamed	1 piece	120	22	4	1

Source: Adapted from Singapore's Health Promotion Board (HPB) website www.hpb.gov.sg. Please check the information obtained from the website as they may have been updated.

The personal trainer can help clients improve carbohydrate intake in their daily meals by encouraging the client to determine the daily amount of carbohydrates needed, convert into number of carbohydrate portions, and make nutritious carbohydrates the core of the diet.

8.4.2 *Protein*

Protein is essential for normal growth and development, the repair and building of muscle tissues, and the maintenance of a good immune system.

Table 8.6. Estimated recommended amounts of protein for various exercise levels.

Group	Recommended Protein Intake (g/ kg/day)	E.g. for a 50 kg person
Sedentary People	0.8 – 1.0	40 - 50
Average Individuals	1.0 – 1.2	50 - 60
Endurance Athletes	1.2 – 1.4	60 - 70
Strength Athletes	1.6 – 1.7	80 – 85

The table above shows the recommended amounts of protein for various exercise levels. The trainer should note that protein requirements for the general population are slightly lower than that of athletes and physically active individuals.

While training does increase the need for protein, most individuals do not have difficulties eating adequate amounts of protein foods especially when they are already consuming a healthy balanced diet. Vegetarian exercisers may need proper planning to obtain good quality sources of protein.

Protein foods are also important sources of minerals including iron, zinc, calcium and B vitamins. There are 2 types of proteins – complete and incomplete. Complete proteins contain all the amino acids (building blocks of protein) for building muscle mass. The best sources of complete protein foods include lean meats, skinless poultry, fish, eggs, low fat dairy products, and soybean products (including tofu and soybean milk). In contrast, plant proteins (with the exception of soybeans) are incomplete proteins. To obtain the complete set of essential amino acids, vegetarians need to eat a wide variety of foods such as dried beans and lentils, rice, bread, cereals, and nuts and seeds.

Many people believe that consuming large amounts of proteins above the recommended amounts is necessary to build bigger muscles. The personal trainer will need to explain that this is not so. The way to build muscle mass is to strength-train correctly while consuming the recommended amount of protein and calories for appropriate exercise level.

Consuming excessive protein foods can lead to dehydration (due to increased fluid loss by the kidneys trying to get rid of waste products from digesting protein), duboptimal glycogen stores (from displacing carbohydrate foods), unnecessary weight gain (from additional fat and calories), and increased calcium excretion in the urine (and possibly contribute to osteoporosis).

8.4.3 *Fats*

Fats are an important source of energy. Fats provide essential fatty acids and fat-soluble vitamins for the body. It is interesting to note that the recommended amounts of fat intake for a normal person and for the physically active individual are the same.

Almost all cuisines use some form of cooking oil when preparing meals, palm oil being one of the most commonly used types of oil in homes as well as in hawker centres in Singapore. Although palm oil is "cholesterol-free", it is high in saturated fat. A high intake of saturated fat can contribute to heart disease by raising blood cholesterol. It is better to use a poly- or mono-unsaturated oil such as canola or sunflower oil. However, research has strong evidence to suggest that olive oil may make the best healthy choice. Nutrition experts recommend a low fat diet of 25-30% of total energy intake coming from fats with the majority of fats coming from unsaturated fat.

Here are some practical tips to reduce fat intake when eating out:

- ❖ Trim and remove all visible fat and skin from meat and poultry, even before cooking where possible.
- ❖ Choose lean cuts of meats.
- ❖ Eat less ribs and fatty meat, chicken wings and processed meat products such as hotdogs and sausages.
- ❖ Minimise foods with coconut milk, pastries and deep-fried foods.
- ❖ Choose low- or non-fat milk and milk products (cheese and yoghurt).
- ❖ Use unsaturated fat cooking oil.
- ❖ Control the amount of oil by preparing most of your own meals.
- ❖ Use low-fat cooking methods such as stir-frying or pan-frying with little oil, steaming, boiling, braising, microwaving, or baking.

8.4.4 *Vitamins and minerals*

In general, if your clients eat a wide variety of foods as part of a well-balanced diet, their vitamin and mineral requirements can be met adequately. However, if your client is a vegan (vegetarians who do not eat any animal products including dairy products or eggs), he/she may require additional supplementation such as vitamin B12 or multi-vitamin and mineral supplements depending on the advice given by a qualified medical professional or dietitian. Section 8.6.1 below provides more information in this area.

8.5 Understanding Hydration

Sweat losses can amount to 1-2 L/hour during exercise, perhaps even more in hot and humid weather. Progressive dehydration from failing to replace sweat losses during exercise has been shown to significantly decrease performance.

Severe dehydration can be life threatening. Warning signs of dehydration include headache, light-headedness, fatigue, irritability or inability to concentrate or pay attention, loss of appetite, dry tongue and lips, dark, concentrated and/or little urine, and frequent muscle cramps.

8.5.1 *Fluids on a daily basis*

Most physically active people need to drink at least 10-12 cups (2.5-3.0 L) of fluids per day. Thirst is not a sensitive indicator of fluid needs during exercise. On a daily basis, fluids include water, milk and malted milk drinks, juices, clear soup or broth, soft drinks, sports drinks, tea and coffee.

Fluids with diuretic effects can lead to dehydration. Be mindful of excessive ingestion of caffeine–containing beverages such as strong tea, coffee and cola drinks. Alcoholic beverages should also not be consumed before, during or after exercise.

Table 8.7. General ways to monitor hydration status.

Monitor the colour of the urine	❖ Drink enough to maintain clear, pale yellow urine throughout the day. ❖ Note that some vitamin supplements (especially vitamin B complex) may turn the urine bright or dark yellow.
Determine sweat loss by weighing before and after training	❖ Aim to replace the fluid loss as quickly as possible. ❖ It may also be useful to work out rates of sweat loss for particular types of exercise sessions and in different climate conditions (e.g. running in air-conditioned gym versus outdoor track).

8.5.2 *Fluids during exercise*

For exercise lasting 30-60 minutes, drinking 10-12 cups (2.5-3.0 L) of fluids will be mostly adequate. However, for longer exercise sessions, a general guideline of fluid intake of 150-300 ml at regular intervals (e.g. every 15-20 minutes) during exercise will be good.

There is a need to plan for regular drink breaks during exercise sessions. Core body temperatures will rise during exercise, putting clients at higher risk for heat stress if not monitored carefully. Some individuals do not like to drink plain water. Thus, providing palatable drinks and regular drink breaks are keys to keeping clients well hydrated.

For exercise lasting up to 60 minutes, water is recommended as the most common and suitable fluid for rehydration. For longer periods of exercise, fluids containing electrolytes and carbohydrates, such as sports drinks, are best fluids to consume as they are quickly absorbed and provide some energy for working muscles.

Sports drinks are formulated with 20-40 mg sodium per 100 ml and 6-8% carbohydrate by volume (i.e. 6-8 g carbohydrate per 100 ml) for ideal absorption and utilization by the body during exercise. Drinks higher in carbohydrate concentration, such as soft drinks and fruit juices are unsuitable during exercise, and are best taken 3-4 hours before, or after, exercise, if at all.

8.5.3 *Fluids after exercise*

Exercisers should start replacing fluid loss immediately after training. Complete fluid and electrolyte balance within the body is a process that can take more than 12 hours. Sodium chloride also needs to be replaced and this is usually done by eating meals.

8.6 **Dietary Supplements and Ergogenic aids**

Nutritional supplements can be classified into dietary supplements and nutritional ergogenic aids. Dietary supplements are often incorporated into the diets to meet nutritional demands due to training. These include the consumption of sports drinks, sports or nutritional bars, and liquid meal supplements where necessary.

8.6.1 *Multi-vitamin and mineral supplements*

Most of an individual's vitamin and mineral needs can be met when adequate calories are consumed in daily main diets. However, with busy work and conflicting schedules, this may not always be the case. Recent research has shown that people who are physically active may likely benefit from taking a daily multi-vitamin/mineral supplement. If unsure, go for a clinical test by a medical professional or a proper nutritional analysis by a certified dietitian. A second opinion should be able to confirm if there is a genuine need for such intake. Unless there is evidence of a nutrient deficiency, individual nutrient supplementation has not been shown to enhance performance.

Here are few pointers regarding multi-vitamin and mineral supplements:

* ❖ Choose a reputable brand and refrain from purchasing from unknown or unreliable source over the internet.
* ❖ Check that the levels of nutrients on the labels do not exceed the Recommended Dietary Allowance (i.e. not more than 100% of Daily Values).
* ❖ Check the expiry date, buy as needed and do not "stock up" too far in advance.
* ❖ Consult the pharmacist, dietitian/nutritionist or doctor (not retail sales staff) about the effects of the supplements if you have concerns or are unsure of any product.

8.6.2 *Ergogenic aids*

Let's make this clear – trainers and clients should always consult with doctors, qualified sports physicians and/or dietitians prior to taking any ergogenic aids. Ergogenic aids are substances that are claimed to directly improve work output and/or exercise performance. Many of these claims are not supported by scientific studies, and many act only as placebos. The ergogenic aid supplement industry may not really be well regulated, hence clients ought to be aware that what they buy may contain very little of the active substances.

8.6.2.1 *Creatine*

Creatine, in the form of creatine phosphate, supplies most of the energy used by muscles for short bursts of intense work (such that required in weight lifting, sprinting, and tennis serve). When creatine stores in the muscles are depleted, energy can no longer be supplied at the rate required for this intense work. The human muscle has a limit as to how much creatine can be stored.

A naturally occurring compound found in meat and fish, it is available in powder and pills. Creatine supplements will likely be of little benefit to athletes with already high concentrations of muscle creatine or to someone ingesting high doses of creatine for many weeks.

Regarding creatine supplements intake, take note of these additional advice and guidelines:

❖ Generally for loading: 20g (4 x 5g doses) for 5 days; maintenance: 2g/day.

❖ Increased muscle creatine levels result in greater capacity to maintain power output during high intensity exercise, especially in repeated bouts of exercise with little time for recovery.

❖ As excess creatine cannot be stored in muscle and must be excreted by the kidneys, the maintenance dose should not exceed 5g daily.

❖ Vegetarians tend to have lower stores of muscle creatine and demonstrate a greater uptake of creatine after supplementation than those who eat meat.

❖ Creatine does not improve endurance exercise but is associated with an increase in body weight of about 1-3 kg. Initial weight gain is water, but in the long term, the gain might be muscle mass.

❖ Reports of side effects are anecdotal, such as athletes having muscle strains and pulls, or suffer dehydration problems while taking creatine supplements. Athletes who exercise in hot, humid environments and those under-hydrated are at risk of these effects.

❖ The safety of long-term use among children has not been extensively tested.

8.6.2.2 *Caffeine*

Caffeine is thought to improve sports performance through stimulation of adrenaline, the central nervous system and the use of fat for energy production thus conserving glycogen stores. Regarding caffeine as an ergogenic aid, here are some considerations to take note:

- ❖ The physiological response to caffeine is not consistent for all. Some athletes benefit at doses of 6.5 mg/kg body weight (390 mg for a 60 kg person) before endurance exercise, but others respond poorly and suffer decreases in performance.
- ❖ Caffeine, about 30-100 mg per serve, is typically found in tea, coffee, and cola drinks already.

8.6.2.3 *Anabolic agents*

A group of drugs that is probably one of the most commonly abused drugs in the sports and fitness industry. 'Anabolic' means growing or building. Anabolic steroids are synthetic derivatives of testosterone, a natural male hormone. These drugs are also referred to as androgenic steroids.

Testosterone is produced in the testes of the male (2-10 mg/day) and in the adrenal glands of females. The hormone's effects include retention of nitrogen (promoting muscle growth), development of male reproductive system during puberty, growth of body hair, deepening of the voice, and involvement in the developmental changes in muscle, bone structure and density. Athletes using steroids in sports, which can be administered by injection or taken orally, may believe that it gives them some kind of a "winning edge".

In personal training contexts, administering anabolic agents with your client will not be necessary at all. Exercisers need to exercise wisdom – If the product sounds too good to be true, it may be possibly prohibited. Please exercise sound judgment and be aware of the possible adverse effects on health and wellbeing. Here are some further information:

❖ Many nutritional supplements marketed for sport use may contain nandrolone and testosterone precursors. But in many countries, nutritional supplements are not tightly regulated or controlled and these substances may not even appear on the product information.

❖ The side-effects of anabolic androgenic steroids are serious, particularly from long-term use or high dosage. In general, it can lead to water retention which may be a major contribution to the initial weight gain, cardiovascular disease resulting from build up of fat and cholesterol in blood vessels, jaundice, liver cancer, and acne.

❖ In children and adolescents, substance abuse can lead to growth stunting, the result of disturbance of normal bone growth and development.

❖ In women, substance abuse can lead to growth of facial hair, hoarsening or deepening of the voice which may be irreversible, reduction in body fat, menstrual irregularities, male-pattern baldness, prominent musculature and veins, and loss of breast tissue.

❖ In males, substance abuse can lead to reduced sperm production due to suppression of natural testosterone secretion, and increased risk of prostate cancer.

8.6.2.4 *Human growth hormone (hGH)*

Human growth hormone (hGH) is produced by the pituitary gland in the brain and is obviously necessary for growth and development in humans. In medical use, regular synthetic hGH injections are used before the end of puberty to treat inadequate growth hormone secretion in dwarfism. Some doctors do administer hGH injections to reverse the loss of lean muscle mass in the elderly. In adults, the role of hGH and its effect on fuel usage and storage is more complex and there is still a need for more research to be done in this area. Here are some further information:

❖ In sports, abusers generally use hGH to increase muscle mass and strength, increase lean body mass, improve the appearance of the body builder's muscles, making it more "sculpted", and increase adult height in children to maximise their athletic potential where height is an advantage.

❖ Possible side-effects in adolescents include gigantism which means development far above average adult height with enlarged limbs and internal organs.

❖ Side-effects in adults will vary and these include enlarged internal organs, especially the heart which may lead to heart failure, acromegaly (abnormal growth of bones of hands, feet and face), thick and coarse skin, impaired glucose tolerance which may lead up to diabetes, elevated blood cholesterol levels, and possibly premature aging and death.

8.6.3 *What all trainers should ask*

If there are clients who are considering taking supplements or ergogenic substance, the trainer should ask the following questions before recommending or suggesting any usage:

❖ Is it a banned substance?
❖ Who produced them? How was it produced?
❖ Is there any short or long term health risk associated with taking it?
❖ Does the client know about possible adverse health and wellbeing consequences?
❖ What does the substance claim to do?
❖ Is the claim backed by scientific fact?
❖ Is it worth risking?

8.7 Principles of Effective Weight Management

Losing weight and gaining weight is very much about balancing food intake (energy consumed) with the energy demands of the body. When more food energy (calories) is consumed than what the body can use (in physical activity), weight increases. In turn, weight is lost when the body uses up more energy than food consumed. However, weight management is more than the mathematics of balancing calorie consumption and expenditure. Genetics play an important role as well and is an active area of research.

8.7.1 *Weight loss*

Consuming more calories than daily energy expenditure causes athletes to gain unwanted body fat. Although excess calories can also come from consuming too much carbohydrate or protein foods, they are more likely to come from consuming too much fat. Weight can creep up if food intake is not reduced accordingly. Another contributor of calories is excessive alcohol intake (more than 1-2 drinks/day). Calories from alcohol often accumulate as fat in the body.

Here are some helpful tips for losing unwanted body fat:

- ❖ Aim for a gradual weight loss of 0.5-1.0 kg per week. Faster weight loss can result in losing valuable muscle mass.
- ❖ Continue to eat a well-balanced diet. Choose foods high in fibre. They are bulkier, take longer to chew, giving your body time to feel full.
- ❖ Avoid skipping meals. Eat substantially during the day, yet have a lighter dinner. Do not allow the body to starve as it often leads to overeating at the next meal.
- ❖ Be prepared with nutritious snacks such as fruit (fresh or dried), yoghurt, milk, wholemeal bread, wholemeal crackers with low fat cheese, cereal, or vegetable sticks.
- ❖ Clients don't have to purposely abstain from favourite high-fat snacks and foods. This often backfires into a period of overeating on them. Clients may still include them as an occasional treat and/or learn to enjoy them in small portions.
- ❖ Include longer periods of low-intensity exercises (e.g. jogging, swimming, cycling) to help use the body's fat stores.
- ❖ Monitor body fat levels every 2-3 months as a more reliable way of losing fat rather than a change in weight on the scales checked on a daily or weekly basis.

8.7.2 *Weight gain*

Increasing muscle mass for greater strength, power and size is advantageous for individuals, particularly athletes if the sports require it. However, gaining weight can be difficult for some. Some factors that impede muscle mass gain are insufficient energy (calorie) intake, inappropriate weight training and limited genetic potential. Energy demands by the body can be very high during training and periods of growth and development, especially in adolescents.

Some individuals make the mistake of increasing fat intake (so as to increase calorie consumption) and find themselves gaining body fat instead of muscle mass. Here are some helpful tips for increasing weight:

❖ Eat a well-balanced diet high in carbohydrates, low to moderate in fat, and adequate in protein.
❖ Try eating according to the time and not rely on the appetite. Missing meals, especially breakfast and lunch, and skipping snacks mean missing calories and important nutrients to support weight gain.
❖ Maximise energy intake with nutrient-dense food and drinks.
❖ Liquid meal supplements can be used as milk drinks between meals.
❖ Have nutritious snacks easily available at home or in the office.
❖ Engage in appropriate strength training.

8.8 Common Eating Disorders

Anorexia nervosa (AN) and Bulimia nervosa (BN) are two of the most common eating disorders that affect mostly adolescents, young adult women, and some males. In most cases, preoccupation with weight is a primary symptom.

Eating disorders among physically active individuals can be difficult to identify. Signs may include the tendency for excessive training, increased frequency of injury, restrictive eating patterns, frequent self-weighing, and extreme worry over body size and shape.

Table 8.8. Two of the most common eating disorders.

Eating Disorder	General Description
Anorexia nervosa	• Intense fear of gaining weight or growing fat. • Distorted view or perception of own body size, body weight and/or body image. • Tend to either consistently restrict food, or restrict and then binge and purge. • Drastic weight loss over short periods of time.
Bulimia nervosa	• Bingeing on enormous amounts of food and then inducing vomiting to prevent weight gain. • Misusing medications (e.g. laxatives, diuretics or enemas). • Fasting habits. • Could be exercising excessively.

Individuals with eating disorders tend to follow strict dietary rules and often experience guilt and self-condemnation if they break any. These individuals also tend to limit their own intake of what they perceived as "bad foods" and usually will choose low- or non-fat foods. Some may even claim to be vegetarian to hide their food limitations.

Very often, individuals with eating disorders also suffer from low self-esteem and an inability to cope with the stresses of life. They will require a sensitive but firm approach to seek help from medical or counselling professionals trained in this area. The treatment of eating disorders will require a multidisciplinary team approach that includes the doctor, psychologist or psychiatrist, nutritionist or dietitian, and trainer.

If the trainer suspects a client who may have an eating disorder, here are general practical steps to consider:

❖ Approach the client with genuine concern, not accusingly, and express your concerns about his or her health and performance. Avoid mentioning about starving or bingeing behaviours in your conversations.

❖ Provide evidence to show why you believe the client may be struggling to balance eating with exercise. Ask if he or she would like to talk about it with you, a trusted friend or family member, or with a counsellor.

❖ If the client opens up to you, try to talk in suggestion of your willingness to accompany him or her to seek professional help in the first instance.

❖ Be patient and supportive. Listen empathetically. Affected individuals are often in denial.

❖ Speak to other trusted people (family member, counsellor, pastoral care, or medical professional). The trainer should not try to deal with it alone.

❖ Organise a sports nutritionist or dietitian to speak to the client about nutrition where appropriate.

8.9 Action Strategies

Shopping assignment – identify hidden or misleading messages in marketing strategies and food labels. Work out plans for wise and healthier food choices. Check out the world's multi-billion food industry in health foods, organic choices, supplements, etc., and try to understand the 'power' of media selling.

Try discussing with family members, friends, and people close to you about this. You might find varying perceptions on this matter. Highlight what tempt people to make certain choices, understand what drives decisions in most consumers, and what makes healthy decisions difficult for consumers. Subsequently work out a plan to educate your clients on such matters with the aim to influence and inspire a more balanced outlook on such matters.

8.10 Summary and Key Points

In this business, we should not underestimate the importance of the roles and responsibilities of the personal trainer in the nutritional education department. Many times, the trainer can create and influence in the client the right mental model towards healthy eating and maintaining a well-balanced body weight and lifestyle. In reality, it is possible to gradually make successful transition to healthy food choices by clients in small steps, which in turn can bring satisfying rewards.

8.11 Recommended Readings and Website Resource

(1) Antonio, J. and Stout, J.R. (2002). *Supplements for Strength-Power Athletes*. Human Kinetics, USA.

(2) Burke, L. and Deakin V. (2000). *Clinical Sports Nutrition*. 2nd Ed. McGraw-Hill, USA.

(3) Chia, M., Leong, L.L. and Quek, J.J. (2004). *Healthy, Well and Wise: Take PRIDE for a Life of Wellness*. National Institute of Education, Singapore. Order details: Office of Graduate Programmes and Professional Learning.

(4) Wolinsky, I. and Driskell, J.A. (2004). *Nutritional Ergogenic Aids*. CRC Press, USA.

(5) Developed by a team of sport specialists from the National Institute of Education, SSSS is a scientific and holistic approach to understanding and practising the principles of science for conditioning for health and fitness. SSSS will help clients get the most out of their sporting pursuits, training, practice or competition: www.sportsuccess.nie.edu.sg

(6) http://www.mayoclinic.com is an award-winning consumer Web site that offers health information, self-improvement and disease management tools. This website contains relevant health and fitness related resources such as healthy living articles, videos and slide shows that fitness professionals will find useful.

(7) Check out this website: www.hpb.gov.sg. The Health Promotion Board of Singapore provides good weblinks and useful articles on nutrition issues relevant to this chapter. There are good data on Asian-related foods as well.

Chapter 9

Individualising Programme Design

It is important for personal trainers to be able to individualise according to unique needs and requirements of clients, especially those with special needs and/or those who are high-risk.

One of your successes as a personal trainer is reflected by your client reaching a point where he or she is comfortable with the changes in his or her physical self and lifestyle. Maintenance of health and fitness will eventually become an important, rewarding and exciting time of the rest of your client's life.

After completing this chapter, you will be able to:

❖ Understand, adapt and modify programmes in relation to individuals' basic 'likes' and 'dislikes'.

❖ Assess fitness using common tests, including the 6-min walking test for elderly, and PWC_{170} cycle ergometer test for overweight individuals.

❖ Understanding general blood pressure status.

❖ Understand programme considerations for special cases such as overweight, elderly, asthmatics.

❖ Recognise signs and symptoms of overtraining and response accordingly.

❖ Understand referrals and levels of readiness to help effect and maintain healthy lifestyle choices.

9.1 Clients Have Unique Needs

Not everyone understands their own perceptions and decisions to exercise and healthy lifestyle, all of which can be easily influenced by many factors. However, every individual will have personal needs, if not

153

'health and fitness' needs. The personal trainer ought to try to understand common reasons people give for not wanting to exercise or participate in healthy activities before attempting to design any exercise training programme for clients.

Habit remains the single best predictor of inactivity across all age groups. Adults particularly need to overcome a lifetime of ingrained behaviour. Trainers are in a good position to impact and influence exercise beliefs of clients. Often, trainers need to match their advice to the client's perception of how physical activity may be beneficial (e.g., weight loss, improved fitness, reduced coronary risk) and build on their individual beliefs to effect a positive change in behaviour. In this way, goals set will avoid the discouragement of unrealistic expectations.

Understanding common barriers to exercise will put personal trainers on the upper hand of matters:

Table 9.1. Possible barriers and what the trainer can do.

Habit	Incorporate activities into daily routine. Give lots of encouragement. Promote active lifestyle gradually.
Self-efficacy	Emphasis is on success for the individual. Begin slowly with exercises that are easily accomplished and advance gradually. Keep track and made known of these small successes. Give frequent encouragement.
Attitude	Promote more positive personal benefits of exercise. Identify enjoyable activities perceived by the client.
Discomfort	Vary intensity and range of exercise. Keep training varied and employ cross-training approaches. Avoid overdoing.
Fear of Injury	Build up balance and strength first. Use appropriate clothing, equipment, and provide supervision. Start slowly and gradually increase in activities and intensity of exercise as client gains confidence.
Disability	Specialised exercises; consider physical therapist or a professional trained in this aspect of disability.
Subjective Norms	Identify and recruit significant or influential others as perceived by the client. May take a while to convince and educate these significant or influential family and friends.
Low Income	Planning for activities may cost quite a bit. If cost is the concern, choose activities such as walking, swimming, ball games on the open field and other simple exercises may be more acceptable to the client.
Environmental Factors	Incorporate activities into client's lifestyle. Walk faster in shopping mall, make use of stairs, park at a further carpark, and make use of community clubs. Exercise indoors when outdoor weather is not ideal.

Illness or Fatigue	Use a range of exercises or intensities that clients can match to their varying energy level. Don't have to work out 'hard' all the time. When experiencing fatigue, go for a gentle walk instead of a jog.
Cognitive	Keep exercises simple. Instructions must be simple and short. Will have to repeat instructions very often. Incorporate into daily routine.
Distractions	Allow clients to choose the activities they think they might enjoy better. Emphasis is on fun, enjoyment, and other benefits including social enjoyment. Provide incentives that can be rewarded across shorter periods of time. Track and make known small successes to client.
Time	Keep the duration of activities short and effective. Choose exercises that are of moderately high intensity to provide a good workout. Exercise at venues convenient to them most importantly. Keep them varied to maintain motivation and enjoyment. Incorporate activities into lunch time hour, or other available free slots throughout the day.
Personality	Depending on individuals. Group exercise class for clients who are extroverted. A small group, one-on-one, or home programme for those who are more introverted.

9.2 Theoretical Models that Explain Lifestyle Changes

Sometimes, understanding stages of change and theoretical models that explain lifestyle changes can help to promote a range of positive behaviours in clients.

While trainers typically have many ideas of what are correct and right to do, clients may not always see in the same light. The main idea of the Transtheoretical Model is that doing the correct things at the right time (stage of change) is important to self-change in health behaviours. Try to identify what's happening or is important to your client during that frame of time in order to customise a programme that seems appropriate and right to do at that time.

The Self–Determination Theory emphasises intrinsic motivation and making personal choices rather than allowing external pressures to determine choices. When working with the client, the trainer could highlight the importance of choice in a person's life and draw out the client's perception of how competent he or she can be in mastering life's tasks. At some points of the programme, the trainer could provide opportunities to the client the autonomy to choose what, when and how to do some aspects of the programme and explain his or her choices.

Both Theory of Reasoned Action and Theory of Planned Behaviour have some similarities. The Theory of Reasoned Action says that the person's behaviour is linked to the person's intention to do that behaviour, and the person's intention is likely most influenced by attitudes (i.e. own beliefs) and social environment (i.e. others' opinions).

The Theory of Planned Behaviour, when combined with Theory of Reasoned Action, adds the concepts of "perceived control" over the environment. In the personal training context, allow the client to believe he or she has some control over the factors that allow performance of that behaviour, and not always be subjected to enforced beliefs and opinions of others and the social environment, including those of the trainer.

The Social Cognitive Theory, also known as 'Social Learning Theory', emphasises self-efficacy and positive expectations about behaviour change. It suggests that for a person to change behaviour, he or she must first value the outcomes of that behaviour. Create opportunities to discuss and debate over various outcomes of lifestyle behaviours with your client. Where the client's views differ greatly and sway from optimal perspectives, remain open to the views and opinions of the client, yet tactfully provide reasonable alternative views for the client to ponder upon in contradictory circumstances.

The Health Beliefs Model states that the person's health behaviour is related to 5 factors: (a) belief that health problem will have harmful effects; (b) belief that one is susceptible to the problem; (c) perceived benefits of changing one's lifestyle to prevent the problem; (d) perceived barriers to overcoming problem; (e) confidence to do the necessary to prevent it. Once again, in any personal training context, plenty of opportunities will surface for open dialogue and discussion of health problems and ways of preventing them between the trainer and client.

The Social Ecological Model states that health behaviour change is influenced by the interaction of intrapersonal, social, cultural, and physical environmental factors. Dialogues and discussions with the client do not always have to focus on self-related issues. At times, the trainer could also discuss with the client the efforts of the public health sectors and the importance of the multitude of social and environmental factors on public health to build a more meaningful and holistic intellectual understanding of health and wellness at large.

9.3 The Meaning of Maintenance

Maintenance is about reaching or achieving a certain health or fitness level a trainer has identified with the client that allows the client to be comfortable with the changes in his or her physical self and lifestyle.

After any amount of sustained training, usually over several months or more, a slow-down in training benefits may be evident. It is at such a point that constant pushing and pressure imposed on the client may cause the client to develop a sense of failure to meet previously set goals.

The trainer needs to prepare the client of this inevitable physiological phenomenon so that he or she can experience it in a positive manner. The trainer could sit down with the client as a unique educational opportunity and explain these issues to the client with the aim of helping the client understand the reasons and need to readjust previously set goals and expectations. From here, new goals and expectations could target generic lifestyle issues that can affect the client's long-term quality of life rather than specific fitness issues.

9.4 Assessing Fitness

Trainers can assess clients' physical capacities periodically at different stages of the programme, particularly prior to the beginning of the programme, every two to three months onwards, and again at the end of the programme.

Collecting information from a battery of fitness tests is useful to both the trainer and the client. It allows the trainer to assess the levels of improvement made, as well as the physical strengths and weaknesses of the client at that stage of training. Results from testing can be used to motivate the client and provide feedback for the way ahead. The trainer can also monitor the client's progress throughout the programme more objectively.

9.4.1 *Principles of testing*

It is important that the trainer understands the basic principles of testing. There are testing procedures that must be adhered to regardless of the choice of the testing protocols or whether the test is conducted in the laboratory or field settings. The trainer must make time to discuss with the clients the need and usefulness for testing, and above all, the reasons for wanting to perform certain testing on them, and what will be involved throughout the whole process of testing.

Some of the points for discussions with the client may include:

- ❖ Identify existing strengths and weaknesses.
- ❖ Predict potential performance.
- ❖ Design appropriate or modify programme to suit the client better.
- ❖ Offer objective feedback (not criticism) to the client.
- ❖ Measure and monitor improvement throughout the programme.
- ❖ Assess or evaluate success of the training programme.
- ❖ The return of investment of the client.
- ❖ Motivate the client.

9.4.1.1 *Principle of specificity*

Testing must be specific to the training requirements of the client being tested. The main considerations to be made when choosing suitable tests according to this principle of specificity are (i) the nature of the training, (ii) the fitness and energy requirements for training, and (iii) the muscle groups predominantly used.

9.4.1.2 *Principle of validity*

A test must reflect the training activity in question. For example, a treadmill test would have lower validity for someone who swims for aerobic fitness. When choosing test protocols, make sure the validity of these tests have been established in previous research studies. The trainer should not make up a totally new test that has not been examined before.

9.4.1.3 *Principle of reliability*

A test should consistently reproduce a given result over repeated testing. For example, a running test conducted on dry ground as opposed to testing on a wet ground even though the same test protocol applies will not produce quite the same results. Trainers need to ensure adequate preparation such as types of equipment and testing procedures, as well as check the weather forecast and environmental conditions if the test is to be conducted in the outdoors to ensure reliability of testing.

Some examples of considerations to be made to ensure reliability of testing include examples such as checking that the bicycle ergometer for testing is properly maintained or calibrated before testing, making sure that the test is to be conducted at the same time as previous testing, whether the female client is having menses (which may mean the need to postpone the test), and ensuring adequate hydration.

9.4.2 *The importance of standardisation*

Fitness tests should only be conducted by qualified or accredited trainers or personnel who will know how to properly prepare, maintain calibration and use testing equipment. They also understand proper documentation of testing protocols and procedures. In this way, trainers and clients will be well assured that test results are not only valid and reliable, but also accurate for interpretation.

Testing should be conducted at the same time of the day because of physiological responses vary throughout the day. The trainer ought to enquire the female client on normal menstrual cycle such that the test will not coincide with the week of menstrual cycle.

Testing ought to be conducted within the same time span as previous testing session. Environmental factors to be controlled include temperature, humidity, noise, and even personal factors such as food and fluid intake, and client's mood.

If bad weather occurs, testing can be postponed, or the trainer may conduct the test in a suitable indoor venue, but as long as it does not inconvenient the client. "Bad weather" may be considered as raining, stormy and very windy day.

Warm-up routines must be included prior testing and should be standardised. Provide the same amount of rest periods and number of trials. Motivation given should be consistent and according to the guidelines of the test protocol.

9.4.3 *Preparing client for testing*

Do not assume the client understands the purpose and procedures of testing. Trainers need to explain to their clients the necessary preparation to be made prior to testing. In this way, the client can report to the testing venue in a well-prepared state.

Here are some useful points to take note of for the briefing session with the client to help get ready before testing:

- ❖ No exhaustive exercise the day before and on the day prior to testing so that results will not be affected by residual fatigue.
- ❖ Have plenty to drink the night before and prior to testing.
- ❖ Prepare sufficient water or sports drink on the day of testing.
- ❖ No eating three hours before testing to allow for adequate digestion.
- ❖ Perform standardised warm-up before the physical testing.
- ❖ Come in proper attires including appropriate t-shirts, sports-bra if required, exercise shorts or sweat pants, exercise towel, appropriate exercise shoes, etc.
- ❖ What to do in the event of "bad weather".
- ❖ Prepare a list of emergency contacts, important phone numbers, and hospital contacts, etc.

9.5 Common Testing Protocols

Some fitness testing, for example a VO_2max test, conducted in the laboratory may be more necessary for specialised sports purposes, particularly for those in elite sports. However, field-based testing is gaining popularity where clients can be assessed in the same surroundings as they train. Field testing can be easily administered to clients without the need for sophisticated testing equipment and highly trained personnel or specialised expertise.

In this chapter, common laboratory and field-based testing protocols are discussed. Based on the above mentioned principles of testing, the trainer must make appropriate decision to the choice of testing protocols suitable for the client in its context.

9.5.1 *Aerobic capacity*

The two most common methods of aerobic fitness in the laboratory are the maximal oxygen uptake (VO_2max), and the anaerobic threshold (AT) tests, which are discussed very briefly. It is unlikely that trainers would conduct these laboratory tests with the clients in a personal training setting, unless the client is an elite athlete with very specific fitness goals. In which case, the trainer can also refer the client to the Singapore Sports Council or other institutions that provide VO_2max testing facilities and services.

A 3-stage incremental submaximal bicycle ergometer test called the PWC_{170} is introduced here as it is felt that this test, being non-impact, may be more suitable for overweight clients and older clients.

The common field tests for endurance introduced here are the Multistage Shuttle Run Test, also known as the Beep Test, the 12-minute Run/Walk Test, and the 6-minute Walking Test.

9.5.1.1 *Maximal oxygen uptake*

Maximum oxygen uptake (VO_2 max) test is a progressive incremental exercise done either on a treadmill or other exercise ergometers until the subject exercise to exhaustion and can no longer go on at a designated workload.

Exhale breaths are collected via a mouthpiece which the subject wears throughout the test. The purpose is to measure the subject's capacity to absorb oxygen into the blood and utilise it. The VO_2max is considered to have been reached when the oxygen uptake fails to increase despite a further increase in workloads. It is at this point that the athlete is exhausted and cannot continue with further increase in workload.

In weight-supported sports such as cycling and swimming, VO_2max is usually expressed as an absolute figure in liters of oxygen consumed per minute (L/min). Otherwise, it is usually expressed as a relative figure in milliliters of oxygen consumed per minute per kilogram of body mass (ml/min/kg).

9.5.1.2 *Anaerobic threshold*

Lactic acid begins to accumulate in the blood faster than it can be removed once a certain level of aerobic capacity is exceeded even before VO_2max is reached. This percentage of VO_2max is known as the anaerobic threshold (AT). Here, blood sampling is required at the end of each workload while the subject performs the VO_2max exercise test and is analysed for lactic acid concentration.

This test result, when used with other data such as heart rate and oxygen uptake at the anaerobic threshold, can be used to determine more accurately the training zones. Unless the client is a serious athlete who will need to perform regular testing to ensure that training zones are adjusted to produce appropriate physiological responses, this test will not be appropriate in most personal training contexts.

9.5.1.3 *PWC_{170} submaximal bicycle ergometer test*

The submaximal Predicted Work Capacity test at heart rate 170 (PWC170) exercise test on a bicycle ergometer in a laboratory or enclosed indoor settings is recommended for most individuals, particularly those who are overweight or older adults.

The test is 12 minutes in duration and involves 3 consecutive incremental workloads cycling at a cadence rate of 60 revolutions per minute (rpm). Workload for each 4-minute interval is determined according to target heart rate zones.

Heart rate is measured using a heart rate monitor employing the telemetric method. Heart rates for the last 2 minutes of each 4-minute interval is recorded and averaged. A line of best fit (Heart rate, beats per minute (bpm) versus Workload, kgm^{-1}min^{-1}) can then be plotted and extrapolated to obtain the estimated projected workload at a heart rate of 170 bpm.

The test is non-invasive and no special preparation is required by the client. The described PWC$_{170}$ test is currently quite a well established functional capacity test for recent obesity research studies.

9.5.1.4 *Multistage shuttle run*

The multistage shuttle run or beep test is a field test suitable for most healthy individuals, but may be too vigorous for older adults and overweight individuals. It is documented as a valid and reliable test for the estimate of endurance fitness (i.e. predicted VO$_2$ max).

Each shuttle stage is 2 minutes with each stage increasing by 1 MET (about resting oxygen consumption). This test involves a series of 20-metre runs that increase in pace according to protocol's set timing with a beep sounded by a tape recorder. The trainer needs to locate only a 20-metre levelled, unobstructed space, either indoor or outdoor, the required beep tape and a tape player. The client continues running until a point when it is no longer possible to keep in time with the beeps on the tape. Each test usually may take about 12 to 15 minutes to complete.

Although the test provides immediate feedback on performance, the existing norms are based on foreign adult standards, hence may not be suitable for local populations. Performance in the test includes elements of self-paced judgement, and some agility is required in turning swiftly at the end of each shuttle.

Field tests generally can be affected by the motivation of the client as well on the day of testing. Trainers must carefully monitor the client to ensure keeping up in time with the beeps sounded by the tape recorded when making to the 20m line at each end, especially when the pace of running becomes faster.

9.5.1.5 *12-minute run/walk test*

For this field test, subjects are required to cover as much distance as possible within the fixed time period. Both running and walking are allowed. Trainers can administer this test in a housing estate stadium that comes with a fixed track of 400m where possible. Alternatively, trainers can make use of quiet and levelled, unobstructed beach paths or an open housing estate area. Of course, prior planning is required. The route is measured prior and pre-determined distances designated within reasonable supervision views using coloured markers or cones. This is to facilitate recording of total distance completed for this test. The distance is recorded in meters.

Since these tests are self-paced tests, clients can be affected by motivation on the day of the test. As mentioned, the regression equation and existing norms are based on foreign adult standards, hence may not be suitable for local populations. It is possible to use just the total distance covered as the test result and a variable for comparison with future test scores.

9.5.1.6 *6-minute walking test*

The 6-min walk test (6MWT) is commonly used to assess the functional exercise capacity of individuals with some forms of cardiovascular and cardiopulmonary diseases. This test is also appropriate for older adults and overweight individuals.

Recent studies have established regression equations to predict the 6-min walk distance in healthy Caucasian populations but these regression equations have yet to be established for the Singaporean population. The limited published data available on equations derived from Caucasian subjects showed consistent overestimation of the 6-min walk distance for the Asian group.

This test is easy to administer. The trainer needs to find a quiet, straight, unobstructed pathway or along a corridor, approximately 50 meters will do. The purpose is to find out how far the subject can walk in 6 minutes to and fro the starting point and the 50m mark.

The walking route must be flat and pre-determined short distances designated using coloured markers or cones (e.g., every 10m) for easy identification of distances marked out. Total distance completed for this test is recorded in meters. Like the 12-minute run/walk test, the 6-minute walking test is also a self-paced test.

9.5.2 *Tests for flexibility*

Flexibility is typically assessed by measuring the range of motion at the various joints. Assessing the client's flexibility could serve several purposes:

- ❖ Provide information about the client's current level of flexibility.
- ❖ Establish specific training goals for both short and long terms.
- ❖ Monitor changes in flexibility as a result of training.
- ❖ Help to identify areas of weaknesses and possible risk of injury.
- ❖ Motivate client and provide feedback.

There are many ways to measure the client's ROM about a joint. Although flexibility can be measured in a laboratory setting, it will require equipment of varying sophistication. On the other hand, field testing can be easily and simply administered without sophisticated testing equipment. In personal training settings, there are easier field tests that can be carried out quickly at any suitable indoor or outdoor venue.

Here are general guidelines to consider for flexibility testing:

- ❖ Clothing should not be restrictive or too loosely fitted. If the client, regardless of gender, is not comfortable with wearing a bathing suit, which is not peculiar to an Asian culture, it is more appropriate to suggest fitting sleeveless t-shirt and a fitting pair of shorts. For some clients, they might even prefer wearing a pair of long stretchable sweat-pants.
- ❖ Testing is to be conducted without shoes on.
- ❖ Prior to testing, a general 5 to 10 minutes warm-up and gentle stretching will be sufficient to prepare the client and to avoid risk of muscle straining.
- ❖ The client, by personal will, must not attempt to force the body to perform movements beyond limits to the point of pain. By the same token, the trainer should allow the client to have active control of the task on hand, and not provide aggressive encouragement to the client to try harder.

- ❖ The same tests can be conducted every 1-2 months to monitor the client's progress. Results of these tests can be used to prescribe appropriate on-going stretching and complementary strengthening exercises to improve posture and overall flexibility.

This chapter offers some of the most common testing methods for the safe and effective assessment of general posture and flexibility suitable for most of the population. These tests are able to provide good indications of regional flexibility.

Even though the Sit & Reach test remains one of the most popular tests to assess flexibility, and is discussed below, it may not be suitable for some clients. For instance, elderly clients with movement limitations or clients with some degree of lower back problems might experience difficulty in performing the Sit & Reach test properly. Personal trainers are strongly encouraged to explore beyond using just a simple Sit & Reach test measure to assess client's flexibility.

9.5.2.1 *Sit & Reach test*

A general test of lower back and hamstring flexibility. Lower back flexibility is important because tightness or weakness in this area is implicated in back problems such as lumbar lordosis, forward pelvic tilt and lower back pain. Test procedures include:

- ❖ Sit on the floor or mat with legs stretch out straight ahead.
- ❖ Feet (shoes off) are placed flat against the box.
- ❖ Knees should be kept straighten and not be bent during the test.
- ❖ Lean forward slowly as far as possible and hold the greatest stretch for two seconds.
- ❖ Make sure there are no jerky movements.
- ❖ The fingertips remain level and stretched while moving forward.
- ❖ The score is recorded as the distance before (negative score) or beyond (positive score) the toes.
- ❖ Take the best of two or three trials.

9.5.2.2 *Measuring ROM using goniometers*

Joints, or articulations, hold the bones together and allow the rigid skeleton some flexibility so that gross body movements can occur. Every muscle of the body is attached to bone (or other connective tissue structures) at two points at the least, the origin and the insertion. Body movement occurs when muscles contract across the joint. The type of movement depends on the construction of the joint and on the position of the muscle relative to the joint.

There are not many publications on the correlations between performance and flexibility, defined as the range of movement (ROM) about a joint. Nevertheless, flexibility appears to be specific, depending on the nature of the activity. Low levels of flexibility can lead to increase susceptibility to injury while very high levels of flexibility in the joint may predispose to dislocation. This section discusses a field method of flexibility assessment when accurate measures of client's range of motion are not necessary.

The most common instrument used to measure ROM about a joint is the goniometer, which is relatively inexpensive to buy, small in size, light and portable, and very easy to use. The goniometer consists of two arms, a stationary (protractor) and a movable bar (dial), both in clear plastic which permits observation of the joint's axis and range of motion.

ROM is measured in degrees (°), using either a 180° or 360° system. ROM can either be active (moved by the muscles acting on the joint) or passive (moved by an outside force). Passive measurement of ROM may produce slightly greater value.

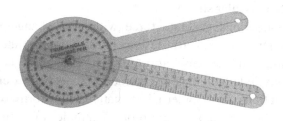

Fig. 9.1. A picture of a universal goniometer.

As shown in the figure below, measuring ROM about a joint can provide some valuable information regarding the client's functional status. A person having difficulty moving about a reasonable range of movement at body joints is likely to experience some degrees of difficulty functioning in their essential daily tasks. For example, having a significant limited elbow flexion may affect the ability to comb the hair or brush the teeth, while severe limited forearm pronation may affect a person's ability to shower, dress up or iron clothes.

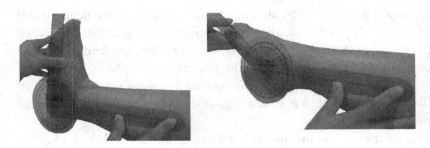

Fig. 9.2. Foot dorsi-plantar (left to right pictures) flexion – using a goniometer to measure ROM at the ankle joint.

9.5.3 *Tests for strength*

There is no one single test for muscular strength. Each strength test is specific to the action and muscle groups being tested. There are various types of muscular contractions and hence different tests to evaluate different types of muscular strength.

Isometric contractions generate force without a change in muscle length (constant length). Isometric testing is most appropriate to assess maximum strength in the laboratory setting. Isoinertial contractions involve either muscle lengthening or contraction (constant external load). Most sporting actions are isoinertial in nature, this form of strength testing can easily be done in a weight room. Examples of testing tasks in the weight room include using the bench press, squat, and leg press, etc.

Isokinetic contractions maintain a constant muscle tension throughout the range of motion (constant tension). Isokinetic strength testing is mainly used where control of joint acceleration is particularly important, for example to determine the effectiveness of an injury rehabilitation programme and the return of limb strength and muscle tension over a range of motion.

While there are strength tests that can be performed in a laboratory setting that require certain specific equipment (i.e. testing grip strength using spring dynamometers; testing dynamic muscular strength using an isokinetic dynamometer), the 1 RM test remains a general test of muscular strength commonly used by coaches and can be easily performed in any gymnasium setting.

9.5.3.1 *1 repetition max (1 RM) test*

The test determines the maximum load one can lift for one complete repetition. General Preparation for this test include warming up thoroughly with light aerobic exercise and at least 10 mins of stretching to all major muscle groups prior, engage the training partner to spot the client.

Here are general guidelines to think about when administering 1RM test:

- Choose a weight that is about 75 % to 80% of the client's 1 RM.
- Perform the exercise (e.g. bench press or leg press) for one repetition only.
- Rest for at least 5 minutes.
- Add only very small increment to the weight and try again.
- The spotter must be next to the client at all times.
- Keep repeating to a weight that cannot be managed anymore. The weight before that is the 1 RM.
- Record that 1 RM weight as the current score for this test. Use this current score to compare with future scores using the same test to gauge improvement in strength.

While the 1 RM test remains a general test of muscular strength in sports testing situations, testing can also be adapted for 3 RM or up to 10 RM for most individuals.

9.5.4 *Tests for power*

Power can be referred as the degree of "explosiveness" with which force can be applied. It defines the ability to produce or exert a maximal force in as short a time as possible. While strength is important for many activities, power is probably of even greater functional significance, especially in sports that require elements of jumping and throwing. Strength and speed are the two components of power (Power = Strength X Speed).

In the personal training context, this may not be a relevant physical fitness test, unless developing power is a specific fitness goal of the client, and the client is subjected to elements of power training in the training programme.

There are simpler power field tests that can be easily administered without much equipment. These field tests include the vertical jump test, standing broad jump test, and the backwards overhead shot put throw test.

General preparation will include a standardised warm up and at least 10 minutes of stretching. It is important to avoid training the day before testing as it can test results due to residual fatigue. These power tests should be performed first in the test battery.

9.5.4.1 *Vertical jump test*

This test aims to measure leg and general anaerobic power. Test procedures include:

- ❖ Dip the fingers in chalk and stand side on to wall.
- ❖ Make a mark on the wall by raising the arm as high as possible without lifting the heels off the ground.
- ❖ The height of the standing reach is recorded.

- ❖ Bending the knees, jump as high as possible without taking a step, marking the wall at the peak of the jump.
- ❖ Record the jumping mark height.
- ❖ Measure the distance between the two marks, and repeat the test two more times. Take the best of three trials.

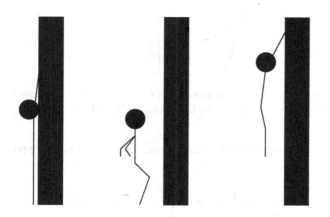

Fig. 9.3. Vertical jump test (adapted and modified from Sports Science in Sporting Success by Chia et al., 2007 with permission).

9.5.4.2 *Standing long (broad) jump test*

This is a test of leg and general explosive power. Test procedures include:

- ❖ Standing at a mark (take-off mark) with feet slightly apart.
- ❖ Swing the arms and bend the knees to jump forward as far as possible.
- ❖ Take off and land with both feet.
- ❖ Make a mark (landing mark) at the back of the heels upon landing.
- ❖ Measure the distance between the two marks, rest and repeat the test two more times. Take the best of three trials.

9.5.4.3 *Backwards overhead shot put throw test*

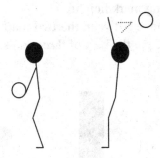

Fig. 9.4. Backwards overhead shot put throw test (adapted and modified from Sports Science in Sporting Success by Chia et al., 2007 with permission).

This test measures upper-body and overall power. Testing procedures include:

- ❖ Use a shot or Medicine Ball (i.e. 4kg for females and 8 kg for males).
- ❖ Face backwards to the field with back of heels on the starting mark.
- ❖ Hold the shot or med ball between the legs.
- ❖ Swing and throw backwards over the head.
- ❖ Stepping past the line for balance after the throw is alright.
- ❖ Measure the distance from the starting line to where the shot or Medicine Ball landed. Take the best of three trials.

9.5.5 *Tests for muscular endurance*

Muscular endurance testing examines the ability of the muscle, or a group of muscles, to resist muscular fatigue and sustain repeated contractions, or to sustain a fixed or static contraction, for an extended period of time.

Muscular endurance can be measured in a number of different ways. For instance, the most popular muscular endurance test in Singapore is to determine the greatest number of sit-ups one can perform in 60 seconds.

Testing can also be done in a weight training room in tasks such as the bench press or leg press by using 50% of 1RM as the resistance.

Other than the sit-up as the most common muscular endurance test in Singapore, other tests of muscular endurance that is appropriate for clients include the maximum number of push-ups in 60 seconds, maximum number of pull-ups one can perform in 60 seconds; or the length of time one can sustain a flexed arm hang. Some of these tests (i.e. sit-up and push-up tests) can even be performed at home.

9.5.5.1 *Sit-up test*

This test measures the overall trunk muscular endurance by simply determining the number of repetitions the client can perform in one minute. Testing procedures include:

- ❖ Start by lying on a mat with hands either across the chest and knees bend.
- ❖ Keep feet flat on the floor.
- ❖ A helper may hold the feet for support.
- ❖ Start the stopwatch to begin the sit-ups.
- ❖ Elbows should touch the knees while performing the sit-ups.
- ❖ Count the number of sit-ups performed in one minute.

9.5.6 *Blood pressure measurement*

Pre-assessment of fitness very often includes the measurement of resting blood pressure. This piece of information is useful for referral should it be discovered that a potential client has indications of abnormal symptoms such as hypertension.

Particularly with obese and elderly clients, it may be necessary to measure the resting blood pressure prior to any exercise session. Other usefulness includes monitoring for dietary changes and improvement of blood pressure in the course of the training programme. Commercial electronic blood pressure monitors are very affordable and easy to use.

The following checks, in addition to the instructions typically provided by the manufacturer, may be applied by the personal trainer when taking a client's blood pressure:

❖ Have the client seated next to a table with musculature relaxed.
❖ The upper arm is bared almost to the shoulder and there should be no constriction due to a tightly rolled sleeve.
❖ If the client is seated instead of lying supine, the forearm is usually placed flat onto the table top with the palm supinated (back of hand touching the table surface) and at the level of the heart. There may be a need to adjust the seat height where appropriate.

9.5.7 *Anthropometry*

Anthropometry is known as the oldest type of body measurement and is used to assess the structure, size and composition of the human body. It is non-invasive and, when done by a trained and experienced anthropometrist, can provide valuable information.

Measurement techniques recommended in this textbook are according to the guidelines of the International Society for the Advancement of Kinanthropometry (ISAK). For the personal trainer, measurements for the 'restricted profile', which is equivalent to the ISAK Level 1 accreditation scheme, comprises of height and weight, eight skinfolds, five girths and two breadths may be well sufficient.

Once the measurement is complete, useful information about an individual is possible by using various computations for data analyses. These may include somatotyping, proportionality estimates, prediction of body density (and subsequently percent body fat) using a number of regression equations, and transformation of the data into age and gender-specific percentile scores for individual sites, overall obesity and proportional mass rankings, as well as other indices such as waist-hip ratio, sums of skinfolds and skinfold-corrected girths.

Minimally, body weight and height, waist-hip ratio, sum of skinfolds, and percent fat mass and lean mass results if available, can provide a good description of the body as a whole. No special preparation is required except that the client wears light clothing for all measures.

Body composition measurements, when made on a repeated basis in the training programme, can provide useful information on the impact of training and dietary programme. Ideally, body composition should be monitored at the beginning of the programme and periodically throughout the programme.

Table 9.2. An example of the ISAK Level 1 - Restricted Profile recording sheet.

Variable	Trial 1	Trial 2	Trial 3	Mean/Median
Height (cm)				
Weight (kg)				
Skinfolds (mm)				
Triceps				
Subscapular				
Biceps				
Iliac Crest				
Supraspinale				
Abdominal				
Front Thigh				
Medial Calf				
Girths (cm)				
Arm (relaxed)				
Arm (flexed and tensed)				
Waist (minimum)				
Gluteal (hip – maximum)				
Calf (maximum)				
Breadths (cm)				
Humerus				
Femur				

Basic testing of body composition usually includes:

- ❖ Height (cm)
- ❖ Body Mass (kg)
- ❖ Body Mass Index (BMI)
- ❖ Sum of Skinfolds (mm)
- ❖ Waist-to-Hip Ratio

It is recommended here that personal trainers interested in employing anthropometry data could contact any of the ISAK Level 3 or 4 Instructors in their local regions for an accreditation course. Refer to the ISAK online website for more information on anthropometry related publications including measurement techniques as described by various authors, and accreditation information (http://www.isakonline.com). The sections below only provide brief information related to the basic testing of body composition.

9.5.7.1 *Height*

Height is measured to the nearest centimetre using a rigid stadiometer. The standard method for measuring height is the 'stretch stature' technique defined as the maximum distance from the floor to the vertex of the head. Height is usually recorded using a stadiometer mounted on a wall with a fixed head piece. The head piece is brought down firmly on the vertex at the same time and the reading taken at this point.

9.5.7.2 *Weight*

Weight is measured to the nearest 0.1kg using a balance scale. Body mass should be obtained on an accurately calibrated beam-type balance or a digital weighing machine. Ideally the subject should be weighed in minimal clothing. The most stable values for monitoring weight change are those obtained routinely in the morning.

9.5.7.3 *Body mass index (BMI)*

BMI is a common measure used by most people. The BMI is computed from the height and weight values in this formula: weight in kilograms divided by height in meters squared.

9.5.7.4 *Skinfold measurements*

The measurement of skinfold thickness can be taken directly below the skin at several specific sites around the body (i.e. biceps, triceps, subscapular, etc.). Measurement of skinfolds should only be done by a skilled ISAK accredited tester. It is necessary to engage a skilled accredited anthropometry tester to administer the measurement of skinfolds to ensure that all measurements are valid and reliable, at the precise landmarks and body sites with repeated measurements. This will ensure accurate comparisons to be made across testing sessions within and between individuals.

Many sports scientists, coaches, trainers and dieticians in Singapore, Australia and around the world are accredited with ISAK. Contact your local ISAK Level 3 or 4 Instructor if you are interested in obtaining ISAK anthropometry certification.

There are some considerations when using skinfold data. For example, the skin and subcutaneous tissue over 3 to 8 standardised sites on the body can be entered into existing regression equations to estimate the percent body fat. To predict percent body fat using regression equations for our population, it will be necessary to develop a set of localised normative database for skinfolds and other anthropometric measurements. Most regression equations commonly used are derived from studies using Caucasian cadavers. Body composition does differ between ethnic groups and also differ between those alive and those dead. As the degree of obesity increase, it also gets harder to pinch a fold of skin to apply the callipers.

Different callipers made by the industry also come with different jaw area and spring pressure. There are many models of skinfold callipers in the market (e.g. Harpenden, SlimGuide, Lange, Lafayette, etc). These callipers vary in jaw pressure (force per unit surface area = $N.mm^{-2}$) which will affect the thickness of the skinfold measurement and the consistency of repeated measurements.

There is currently no standard for either jaw surface area or spring tension. However, two types of callipers, Harpenden calliper and SlimGuide calliper, are currently recognised by the ISAK. Harpenden callipers are currently used as the criterion instrument. In the personal training context, the SlimGuide calliper, which is a much cheaper option, will adequately serve its purpose.

Monitoring intra-individual subcutaneous body fat levels can be achieved by routinely measuring skinfold thickness without further manipulation of skinfold data. A number of skinfold sites are recommended to account for individual fat patterning which can indicate unequal fat loss/gain in specific sites during weight changes. Here, skinfold thicknesses taken over 3 to 8 standardised sites on the body can simply be reported as sums of skinfolds.

9.5.7.5 *Waist-to-hip ratio (WHR)*

The waist-hip ratio (WHR) is computed as waist in unit centimetres divided by hip in unit centimetres. The WHR has been extensively used to discriminate between various types of fat distributions. Waist and hip girths should be measured according to the ISAK guidelines as well. Waist girth is measured at the level of the narrowest point between the lower coastal border and the iliac crest. The client is breathing normally and the measurement is taken at the end of a normal expiration.

The exact location of the waist and hip girth sites may not be straightforward, particularly in the obese group. Where the waist is not obvious, the measurement can be taken at the mid-point between the lower coastal border and the iliac crest. The hip girth is taken at the level of the greatest posterior extension of the buttocks.

Depending on the sites chosen, measured WHR can range widely. Consequently, recommendations about cut-off scores should be interpreted in relation to the measurement sites. Cut-off scores for increased risk have ranged from 0.90 to 1.00 for men and from 0.80 to 0.91 for women. Typically, a WHR in excess of 0.90 for men and 0.85 for women is taken to be indicative of increased risk. For both measurements, the measuring tape should be readjusted as necessary to ensure that it has not slipped and that it does not excessively indent the skin.

9.5.7.6 *Bioelectrical impedance (BIA)*

Since the use of bioelectrical impedance equipment is quite commonplace in gyms and shopping centres, it is worthwhile to make mention of some industry stated scientific values and limitations. BIA equipment usually looks like a complex weighing scale or can just look like a simple hand-held device.

A mild undetectable current is passed through the body between a variable numbers of electrodes embedded within the equipment. The concept of BIA is simple to understand. Muscle conducts the current easily, while fat impedes the current, and thus, the amount of electrical impedance provides an indirect indication of the amount of fat there is in the body.

While BIA appears to be simple to use, there are other variables besides fat and muscle proportion that will affect electrical impedance, such as hydration status. For example, in the first week of weight loss, there is a tendency to lose water in the urine resulting in an overestimation of body fat by BIA. It may also not be accurate enough to detect small changes in weight loss programmes. Measurements taken at different points of the day may also not be reliable.

Most BIA devices also depend on added computation of percent body fat from regression equations that are already preset into the devices. In other words, it is not advisable to monitor daily, weekly or short period of progress using BIA.

9.6 Monitoring Progress

At the beginning of the training programme, the trainer and client should have a clear understanding of their responsibilities for monitoring client's responses to training. It is always good to be well prepared and to device a system to monitor training and recovery on a regular (e.g. weekly) basis. Not all clients respond the same to training. Having a system to monitor progress can allow the trainer to plan activities and workloads to suit the adaptation rates of each client.

There are several recognisable body signs and cues that can be observed as an indication on how the client is coping with training. The trainer can record such observations in a log book. The clients can also perform self-monitoring by recording their responses to training in their own training diaries (i.e. the Client's Training Diary).

Other ways or things trainers can do may include talking with clients and find out how they are doing or coping with training, and observing client's behaviours and body language before, during and after training. Trainers can rely on immediate feedback obtained from resting and exercise heart rates measurements, breathing rates and patterns, as well as observable performance indicators, if any.

9.6.1 *The trainer's observation*

The trainer's observations of the client's adaptation to training ought to include specific signs and cues based on direct communication, client's body language, physiological and psychological indicators and other generic signs and cues such as the eating habits and sleeping patterns.

Table 9.3. An example of a trainer's observations made on a client's responses to training.

Observation Categories	Signs and Cues
Communication issues	• Client said that she felt tired and unable to maintain the pace of jogging throughout
Body language/attitude	• Looked a bit pale • Occasional had bad technique (e.g. slouching and excessive arm swings) when jogging up slopes as compared to normal
Physiological	• Slight increase in resting heart rate in the past three days
Psychological/mood	• Not able to concentrate as compared to normal and constantly felt fatigue and lethargic at work
Others	• Client said that she did not sleep well lately • She also felt not wanting to talk much with colleagues and trainer lately

9.6.2 *Client's training diary*

Clients can be encouraged to keep a training diary so that they can monitor their own training responses to each training session, or at least once a week. This way, clients can learn to listen to their bodies and be able to recognise signs and cues and self-assess on whether they are coping with training or not. Hopefully, this can empower them to properly manage their bodies in and out of training and be responsible towards their own health maintenance and performance.

Possible observations that a training diary can provide include:

❖ The quality of sleep – consistent poor sleep patterns may indicate early signs of overtraining and burnout.

❖ Morning resting heart rate – consistent elevated morning resting heart rates (i.e. 10-12 bpm above usual) is indicative of fatigue or incomplete recovery from previous exercise sessions.

❖ Daily rating of energy levels – feeling tired after training is a normal response, but if the client is feeling constantly tired, it is a sign that the body is fatigue or still adapting to training stressors.

❖ Attitude to training and in general (e.g. work, leisure, etc.) – drastic changes in attitudes and emotions such as feeling irritable easily, or don't feel like going to work may give indications that the client is not coping well.

❖ Others (e.g. communication with others, health, appetite, etc.) – falling sick regularly is indicative of a possible state of overtraining especially if the client is subjected to intense training workloads for quite a prolonged period.

Usually by giving a few days of rest or reduced training is enough for the variables to return to a normal range. However, if there are consistent symptoms of tiredness, poor sleeping patterns for days, and prolonged elevated morning resting heart rates that do not return to normal, the trainer should recommend the client to seek medical advice.

9.6.3 *Self-management skills*

Encouraging the development of useful life skills such as self-monitoring and self-management skills is perhaps the key to successful empowerment for life-long healthy lifestyle.

Table 9.4. Examples of actions for self-monitoring and self-management.

Weekly Actions	Monthly Actions
1. Record resting heart rate before getting busy in the morning for this week. 2. Rate daily energy level at the end of each day before sleeping. 3. Reduce on supper snacks and high-fat diet. 4. Try out the new music album during stretching sessions.	1. Have at least three quality rest days per week this month. 2. Have at least one reduced training day per week this month. 3. Plan at least one active rest for some postural exercises. 4. Organise simple get-together sessions with family and friends on weekends.

Clients can learn how to look after themselves both physically and psychologically. These effective life skills will help clients adapt to regular exercise as an essential part of their lifestyles. Very often, maintenance of such practices requires discipline and time management on the part of the clients, as well as continuous monitoring and giving encouragement on the part of the trainer.

9.7 Action Strategies

Start interviewing people around you, those you know and those whom you are not too familiar with. Find out about what people really understand about 'healthy lifestyle' and what they really want in terms of achieving this. What are the plans and programmes that may work for them?

Interview as many people around you to identify diverse examples of people's 'needs' and 'wants'. Reflect through and critically determine the soundness in these 'needs' and 'wants'. You may find that not all 'needs' and 'wants' are healthy or good for the body. List as many examples of those that are not desirable versus desirable choices in your own trainer's log book for future references as you progress in your career.

9.8 Summary and Key Points

As a personal trainer, you have acquired the necessary knowledge and competence in helping your clients' through their decisions for healthy lifestyle. Your ability to attend to their special considerations is important and is a definite part of the equation to encourage them to sustain healthy living efforts.

9.9 Recommended Readings and Website Resource

(1) American College of Sports Medicine (1998). Position stand on the recommended quantity and quality of exercise for developing and maintaining cardiovascular and muscular fitness, and flexibility in healthy adults. *Med Sci Sports Exerc*, 30, pp. 975–991.

(2) Adams, G.M. (2002). *Exercise Physiology Laboratory Manual*. 4th Ed. McGraw-Hill, USA.

(3) Chia, M., Leong, L.L. and Quek, J.J. (2004). *Healthy, Well and Wise: Take PRIDE for a Life of Wellness*. National Institute of Education, Singapore. Order details: Office of Graduate Programmes and Professional Learning.

(4) Developed by a team of sport specialists from the National Institute of Education, SSSS is a scientific and holistic approach to understanding and practicing the principles of science for conditioning for health and fitness. SSSS will help clients get the most out of their sporting pursuits, training, practice or competition: www.sportsuccess.nie.edu.sg.

(5) http://www.mayoclinic.com is an award-winning consumer Web site that offers health information, self-improvement and disease management tools. This website contains relevant health and fitness

related resources such as healthy living articles, videos and slide shows that fitness professionals will find useful.

(6) ISAK online website: www.isakonline.com. The International Society for the Advancement of Kinanthropometry (ISAK) was founded as an organisation of individuals whose scientific and professional endeavour is related to kinanthropometry. ISAK's purpose is to create and maintain an international network of colleagues who represent the world community transcending geography, politics and the bounds of separate disciplines in order to establish a dynamic area of scientific endeavour.

Chapter 10

Exercise Considerations for Special Cases

Customising programmes will include the importance of correctly assessing client's special status and providing appropriate exercise advice. The ultimate aim should be the sustainability of behaviour change in relation to living with special conditions.

After completing this chapter, you will be able to:

❖ Understand the special conditions of the client.
❖ Understand what the client can and cannot do in terms of exercise requirements in the design of exercise prescription.

10.1 Introduction

The key to success is to know your client's needs and goals, especially those with a special-need and/or those who are high-risk. Some of these common conditions include diabetes, high blood pressure, high blood lipids or cholesterol, obesity, asthma, and the elderly.

It is important for personal trainers to be able to individualise according to unique needs and requirements of clients. As personal trainers are not physicians, it is important to work in concert with the instructions of the physician in functional terms about what the client can or cannot do in terms of exercise. Trainers may also need to know the types of medications that the client is taking and the effects of those medications on exercise responses.

All in all, it is far more important that trainers emphasise the goal of progress and fulfilment. Remember that clients living with special conditions may not be able to perform much, but they can still lead fulfilling, productive and fun-filled lives with exercise.

10.2 Exercise Planning for Managing Obesity

Talks about obesity, its diverse causes and associated health risks, the proposed ways to tackle the obesity problem, reverting back to proper diet and adequate physical activity are common. There is a high chance that personal trainers in Singapore will associate their work in the area of obesity.

Today, planning an exercise programme for this group comes with rather different objectives. The aim is to actively engage them, meet their unique needs and provide support to help them recognise their potential in health and wellbeing. This could mean encompassing different approaches and creative efforts in the training programmes to help these participants cultivate healthy lifestyle habits through diet, sports and games.

10.2.1 *Types of exercises suitable for the obese*

10.2.1.1 *Increase cardiovascular fitness*

Longer duration, low intensity exercises are most appropriate. It is best to choose an intensity that can be sustained for at least 30 to 45 min. Bear in mind that higher impact activities can easily tire or hurt the knee joints. So activities like walking or stationary cycling is advised, as opposed to jogging or running.

To maintain momentum, use a variety or combination of fun activities for cardiovascular fitness and even warm-ups. Ideas could include step aerobics or aerobic dancing, swimming or water aerobics. Try to incorporate game-like activities such as modified drills or practices as much as possible. Regardless of the types of exercise, training sessions could be scheduled at least three times a week.

10.2.1.2 *Increase muscle weight and reduce fat*

Strength-training exercises should be incorporated. However, only simple exercises are advised. Dumbbells may be suitable for obese individuals as certain weight benches and seats of strength machines may be too narrow or small for these participants. Use lighter loads and higher repetitions.

The intensity and duration of the exercise programme should be progressively increased throughout the weeks in accordance with the individual's tolerance level. This should be done by initially increasing the number of exercise circuits from one to three and then by increasing the resistance or cycling load. Aim not for quick results but a gradual increase in muscle mass, which will help increase the participant's basal metabolic rate in the long run.

We recommend circuit strength-training formats for the obese. An exercise "circuit" may also consist of resistance exercises alternated with aerobic stations, such as the stationary cycle or treadmill. The aerobic exercise phases (i.e. 5 to 10 min each) between resistance stations (i.e. total 8 to 10) are designed to maintain the exercise heart rate to facilitate changes in cardio-respiratory fitness and maximise energy expenditure.

All major muscles in the body should be exercised. The whole body training regime should concentrate on the large muscle groups of the lower limbs with selected torso exercises also included.

Two to three sessions per week should be sufficient. Each of these sessions will commence and conclude with at least 10 minutes of warm up/cool down and stretching.

Do note that the obese could have difficulty getting into the supine position, and this may also cause breathing problems. Try to select exercises that do not involve getting up and down from the floor. Avoid squats and lunges as these exercises are difficult for obese individuals, particularly those with knee problems. Obese individuals also may not have good balance to handle these types of exercises.

10.2.2 *Other points to remember*

Most importantly, make your training programme fun and engaging for these clients to keep them coming back for more. This could make a huge impact on their quality of life. Through exercise, personal trainers can play an important role in encouraging obese individuals to develop their confidence and achieve personal goals and a sense of success. Here are some useful pointers:

❖ Obese individuals should consult their doctor or physiotherapist before starting a training programme.

❖ Supervision of obese participants in your programme is essential.

❖ Participants should wear comfortable shoes and loose cotton clothes.

❖ Do not exhaust obese participants. Make training sessions enjoyable for them.

❖ If the individual experiences any breathing difficulty, pain in the chest or other body areas, including the joints, stop the exercise immediately and consult a doctor.

❖ Make sure obese participants drink a lot of fluid as dehydration can occur very quickly.

❖ An air-conditioned training environment is ideal. If this is not available, try to exercise in the shade and avoid training on hot days as obese participants may not dissipate heat as effectively.

10.3 Exercise Planning for Older Adults

Up to 70 percent of older adults over the world are physically inactive. It is well established that regular exercise provides a myriad of health benefits in older adults, and participating in regular physical activity is associated with decreased mortality and age-related morbidity in these individuals.

The importance of promoting geriatric health care at health clubs and senior centres is now widely recognized. Trained geriatric exercise leaders are becoming increasingly common. Exercise prescription for older adults should target aerobic exercise, strength training, and balance and flexibility.

10.3.1 *Types of exercises suitable for older adults*

10.3.1.1 *Increase cardiovascular fitness*

Walking, swimming and water aerobics are considered suitable activities for older adults as these are light, lower intensity activities. Smaller individual bouts of activity such as 3 continuous bouts of 10-minute walks, with periods of brief rest in between are appropriate.

Target a combined total of at least 30 minutes of moderate aerobic activity for most days of the week. Moderate activity corresponds to level walking at a 2.0 to 4.5 mph pace (i.e. 2.5 to 5.5 metabolic equivalents) for most older adults.

Trainers may incorporate aerobic activities into clients' lifestyle early, for example moving the stationary bicycle in front of the television in the living room. Add on to exercises that they are already performing, such as climbing an additional flight of stairs or walking to a further post office each week.

Try to increase intensity by adding more intense activities in daily living first, such as walking up a slope, carry a few bags of goods bought from the supermarket, or increasing arm movements generally in house work, rather than increasing the speed of exercise.

10.3.1.2 *Incorporating strength, resistance training*

Research shows that muscle strength declines by 15 percent per decade after age 50 and 30 percent per decade after age 70. On the other hand, resistance training can result in 25 to 100 percent, or more, strength gains in older adults.

Exercise against resistance or gravity helps to strengthen muscles. Use own body weight as resistance as much as possible. Activities can include floor exercises, weight training, swimming and water aerobics. Not all resistance exercises need to be performed in a gym setting with weight training machines. Incorporate repeated functional activities as much as possible such as reaching forward to a top shelf and rising from a chair can also be effective.

Begin resistance training slowly and gradually work up the intensity of the training regimen. Start with resistive bands or tubing, light weights (e.g. small hand weights or a filled water bottle).

For gym workouts two to three times per week, choose up to eight to 10 different exercises of 10 to 15 repetitions in a set. But start with a manageable number of exercises first and gradually progress up the numbers.

The gym programme should involve all major muscle groups. These include hip extensors, knee extensors, ankle plantar flexors and dorsiflexors, biceps, triceps, shoulders, back extensor, and abdominal muscles. Light weights are good. Each repetition should be performed slowly through a full range of motion.

10.3.1.3 *Improve flexibility and balance*

Deconditioned and sedentary elderly patients should be encouraged to improve their functional ability with strength and balance training before beginning aerobic exercise.

A basic balance exercise programme that incorporates repeated standing on one leg, first with eyes opened, then with eyes closed with progression over time, can help improve stability and may decrease the risk of falls. Such an activity can be done at home. Other basic balance exercises include walking heel-to-toe, and rising to and lowering from a chair.

Only perform exercises at a comfortable level and not be too ambitious in case falling incidences happen while exercising. There must be adequate supervision as balance and postural exercises progress in difficulty.

Supervisions must be present whenever there is a reduction the base of support in one legged stand, unstable center of gravity when performing turns, postural muscles are worked harder in heel raise exercise, and when there is reduction of sensory input when eyes are closed.

Floor exercises combining elements of pilates and calisthenics can be fun. Stretch major muscle groups once per day after exercise when muscles are more compliant. Static stretches are safe and much preferred, and it is advisable to avoid ballistic stretches.

10.3.2 *Other points to remember*

Regardless of the types of exercise planned, keep these pointers in mind:

- ❖ Before initiating an exercise programme, it ought to be made compulsory that all older adults must undergo a history and physical examination directed at identifying cardiac risk factors, exertional signs/symptoms, and physical limitations.
- ❖ Incorporate exercise into a prior routine makes it easier to remember.
- ❖ Keep the exercises simple.
- ❖ Provide specific short instructions and repetition for the learning of new skills.
- ❖ Must have the presence and guidance of a trainer to ensure proper technique and safety. In more complex cases, where medical attention may be required at any time, supervision by a trained geriatric exercise leader, nurse or physiotherapist is necessary.
- ❖ Allow them to choose activities for themselves that they consider enjoyable.
- ❖ Incorporate more social elements (i.e. group activities; fun games) into the design of exercise programme for older adults.
- ❖ If muscles or joints are sore the day after exercising, reduce the activities or intensity of exercise in the next session. Sometimes, an additional day of passive rest may be helpful. But if the pain or discomfort persists, consult the doctor immediately.
- ❖ If any of the symptoms such as nausea, light-headedness or dizziness, chest pain or feeling a compress pressure at the chest area, difficulty in breathing or excessive shortness of breath, extreme difficulty with balance or a sense of poor balance than

usual happen while exercising, stop and consult the doctor immediately.

❖ Wear comfortable shoes and loose cotton clothes, and drink sufficient fluid before, during and after exercise.

❖ An air-conditioned training environment is ideal. Activities conducted at HDB void decks of Singapore housing estates are fine in the mornings and evenings, but avoid activities under direct sunlight.

10.4   Exercise Planning for the Asthmatics

The main reason why most individuals with asthma are staying away from regular exercise and healthy activities as part of their lifestyle is because they are afraid they might experience symptoms when they exercise.

Asthma has several different triggers such as cold air, dust particles or exercise, to name a few. While one person may be able to exercise without a problem, another will find that exercise actually triggers an episode. There are some types of exercise that are better tolerated than others.

10.4.1   *Starting out tips*

Here are some important and useful guidelines for those who wish to start exercising. Before initiating an exercise programme, asthma sufferers should consult a doctor and undergo a physical examination where necessary to find out what types of activities are appropriate, identify exercise limitations and what to do to prevent an episode during exercise.

The presence and guidance of a trained professional may be required for severe asthmatic cases. People with asthma should keep an eye on the weather and pollen counts before exercising. For example, outdoor sports in the cold, monsoon weather may trigger an episode. Activities can be conducted indoors during the cold, monsoon weather.

During exercise, try to breathe through the mouth or through pursed lips instead of breathing through the nose as much as possible. This may not be comfortable in the beginning and may take some time getting used to.

Choose a humid exercise environment. Take a walk or jog on a path near the beach. Swimming is a good activity in this regards. Try to avoid exercise outdoors when air pollution is high.

If an inhaler is prescribed by the doctor, use it before exercising. The doctor will be able to prescribe something that is suitable for the individual. It is necessary to continuously monitor individual progress and exercise at appropriate level. Finally, drink plenty of water, and make sure that the warm-up and cool-down are done slowly without rushing.

10.4.2 *Types of exercise suitable for asthmatics*

Swimming is a very good activity that most people with asthma can tolerate well. The warm, moist air of the swimming pool helps with breathing.

Activities that involve short, intermittent periods of exertion intersperse with breaks in between such as golf, netball, tennis, volleyball and softball are generally well tolerated.

Alternatively, people with asthma usually can also tolerate continuous aerobic exercise such as cycling, aerobics, walking or jogging, as long as the activity is performed at a comfortable pace.

10.4.3 *Types of exercise to avoid*

Try to avoid activities that involve extended periods of exertion as well as activities of very high intensity. These activities include fast paced running, basketball, hockey, heavy weight lifting and long sprints. Stop when the client experience symptoms. For those who can tolerate these sports and games well, it is alright to continue, but do monitor progress and symptoms. It is also wise to avoid participating in activities in cold weather conditions such as ice-skating in an indoor ice-skating ring.

10.5 Action Strategies

Keep informed and updated with the common health ailments that affect the population- young and old. Be knowledgeable about the common medications that are prescribed for those common ailments. Foster good relations with health care practitioners and physicians for appropriate referrals where necessary.

10.6 Summary and Key Points

As a personal trainer, your ability to attend to their special conditions in terms of their exercise needs is important and is a definite part of the equation in encouraging them to lead fulfilling exercise-enabled lifestyles.

10.7 Recommended Readings and Website Resource

(1) American Council on Exercise (1999). *Clinical Exercise Specialist Manual: ACE's Source for Training Special Populations*. In Cotton, R. and Anderson, R. (Eds). ACE, USA.
(2) Chia, M., Leong, L.L. and Quek, J.J. (2004). *Healthy, Well and Wise: Take PRIDE for a Life of Wellness*. National Institute of Education, Singapore. Order details: Office of Graduate Programmes and Professional Learning.
(3) Mazzeo, R.S., et al. (1998). ACSM position stand on exercise and physical activity for older adults. *Med Sci Sports Exerc*, 30, pp. 992-1008.
(4) Wong, P. and Lee, P.C. (2009) Managing obesity in Singapore schools – holistic approaches for the future. In Aplin, N. (Ed) *Perspectives on Physical Education and Sports Science in Singapore – An Eye on the Youth Olympics 2010*. McGraw-Hill Education, Asia.
(5) Developed by a team of sport specialists from the National Institute of Education, SSSS is a scientific and holistic approach to understanding and practising the principles of science for

conditioning for health and fitness. SSSS will help clients get the most out of their sporting pursuits, training, practice or competition: www.sportsuccess.nie.edu.sg.

(6) http://www.mayoclinic.com is an award-winning consumer Web site that offers health information, self-improvement and disease management tools. This website contains relevant health and fitness related resources such as healthy living articles, videos and slide shows that fitness professionals will find useful.

Client Acknowledgement and Indemnity

I, _____ (client's full name) voluntarily choose to participate in a personal training programme that will include weight training and/or cardiovascular and flexibility exercises.

I understand that physical exercise, including the use of all equipment, could be a potentially hazardous activity. I understand that fitness activities involve a risk of injury and even death, and that I am voluntarily participating in the activities and using equipment and machinery with the knowledge of the dangers involved.

I have been informed that to minimise the risk of injury, I should obtain medical approval before participating in any exercise and training programme or using any equipment provided.

I acknowledge that I have either had a physical examination or been given my doctor's permission to participate, or that I have decided to participate in activity and the use of equipment and machinery without the approval of my doctor and assume all responsibility for my participation and activities, and use of equipment and machinery in my activities.

I agree that any information, instruction or advice obtained from personal training is not a substitute for medical treatment or advice.

1 of 2

197

I am aware that I may discontinue participation in the programme at any time that I see fit to do so. I agree that if at any time I experience dizziness, discomfort or pain of any type I will stop exercising immediately and consult a doctor.

I declare that I am physically fit and that I do not suffer from any condition, impairment, disease, infirmity, or other illness that would prevent my participation in the fitness training or use of equipment or machinery.

I assume all risks associated with the exercise and workout programmes and for any physical injury or damage that may arise out of my participation in the training programme or that may result from the use of the training equipment.

I indemnify and hold harmless _____
(full name of personal trainer), consultants, officers, agents and employees of _____
(full name of company) and against all liability, including death and for any claims, demands, actions, loss, and damage arising out of or in any way connected with my participation in the training programme.

Signed_____ (client's signature)

Dated_____

Physical Activity Readiness Questionnaire

This questionnaire is applicable to clients who are below 60 years old and assesses readiness to participate in moderate intensity exercise and above or the readiness to participate in physical fitness tests.

Please tick 'Yes' or 'No' to the questionnaire items	Yes	No
I have a heart condition and my doctor recommends only medically supervised physical activity		
During or right after I exercise, I often experience pain or pressure in my neck, left shoulder, or arm		
I have developed chest pain within the last month		
I tend to lose consciousness or fall over due to dizziness		
I feel extremely breathless after mild exertion		
My doctor recommended that I take medicine for high blood pressure or a heart condition		
I have bone or joint problems that limit my ability to do moderate-intensity physical activity		
I have a medical condition or other physical reasons not mentioned here that might need special attention in an exercise programme		
I am pregnant and my doctor has not given me the OK to be physically active		
I am over 60 years old, have not been physically active and am planning a vigorous exercise programme		
If you answered 'Yes' to one of more questionnaire items, it is important that you see your doctor before embarking on any physical activity or exercise programme.		

Sample Exercise Accounts

Overall Weekly Exercise Summary

Name: _____ Date (week of):_____

Fitness goal: _____
(e.g. build muscle, lose body fat, increase aerobic fitness, flexibility)

Total sleep hours per week:_____

Success of the week:_____

AEROBIC CONDITIONING EXERCISE NOTES

Total sessions	Steps/km	Total hours	Remarks

RESISTANCE TRAINING EXERCISE NOTES

Total sessions	Total repetitions	Total sets	Remarks

FLEXIBILITY TRAINING EXERCISE NOTES

Total sessions	Total number of stretches	Total sets	Remarks

_____
_____

NUTRITION NOTES

Total servings	Rice & alternatives	Meat & alternatives	Fruit	Vegetable	Water

_____
_____

OVERALL WEEKLY WORKOUT RATING
[1 (AWFUL) TO 10 (AWESOME) SCALE]:

_____
_____

NEXT WEEK'S PLAN:

_____
_____
_____

2 of 2

Client's Training Diary

My Training Diary Date: _____
Session No./Week No.: _____/_____
Trainer's Name:_____
Session Objective(s): _____
Session Activities: _____

Observation Categories	Scale 1 to 5 (1 – poorest; 5 – best) Signs and Cues				
Quality of sleep	Circle Comment:	1	2	3	4	5
Morning Resting Heart Rate (bpm)	Circle Comment:	1	2	3	4	5
Daily rating of energy levels	Circle Comment:	1	2	3	4	5
Attitudes about training	Circle Comment:	1	2	3	4	5
Emotions	Circle Comment:	1	2	3	4	5
Communication with people	Circle Comment:	1	2	3	4	5
General health	Circle Comment:	1	2	3	4	5
Appetite	Circle Comment:	1	2	3	4	5
Others	Circle Comment:	1	2	3	4	5

Bibliography

Adams, G.M. (2002). *Exercise Physiology Laboratory Manual.* 4th Ed. McGraw-Hill, USA.

Alter, M.J. (1996). *Science of Flexibility.* Human Kinetics, USA.

American College of Sports Medicine (1995). Osteoporosis and exercise. *Med Sci Sports Exerc,* 27, pp. 1-7.

American College of Sports Medicine (1998). Position stand on the recommended quantity and quality of exercise for developing and maintaining cardiovascular and muscular fitness, and flexibility in healthy adults. *Med Sci Sports Exerc,* 30, pp. 975–991.

American College of Sports Medicine (2001). *ACSM's Resource Manual for Guidelines for Exercise Testing and Prescription.* 4th Ed. ACSM, USA.

American Council on Exercise (1999). *Clinical Exercise Specialist Manual: ACE's Source for Training Special Populations.* In Cotton, R. and Anderson, R. (Eds). ACE, USA.

Antonio, J. and Stout, J.R. (2002). *Supplements for Strength-Power Athletes.* Human Kinetics, USA.

Armstrong, R.B. (1984). Mechanisms of exercise-induced delayed onset muscular soreness: A brief review. *Med Sci Sports Exerc,* 16, pp. 529-538.

Åstrand, P.O. (2003). *Textbook of Work Physiology: Physiological Bases of Exercise.* 4th Ed. Human Kinetics, USA.

Balady, G.J. and American College of Sports Medicine (2000). ACSM's Guidelines for Exercise Testing and Prescription. 6th Ed. Lippincott Williams & Wilkins, USA.

Beard, J. (2002). Iron status and exercise. *Am J Clin Nutr,* 72 (Suppl), pp. S594-S597.

Bergstrom, J. and Hultman, E. (1967). Muscle glycogen synthesis after exercise: An enhancing factor localized to the muscle cells in man. *Nature,* 210, pp. 309-310.

Bloomfield, J., Ackland, T.R. and Elliott, B.C. (1994). *Applied Anatomy and Biomechanics in Sport.* Blackwell Scientific Publications, UK.

Bompa, T.O. (1999). *Periodization: Theory and Methodology of Training.* 4th Ed. Human Kinetics Books, USA.

Borg, G.A. (1970). Perceived exertion as an indicator of somatic stress. *Scand J Rehab Med,* 2, pp. 92-98.

Borg, G.A. (1982). Psychological basis of perceived exertion. *Med Sci Sports Exerc*, 14, pp. 377-381.

Borg, A., et al. (1987). Relationship between perceived exertion, HR and HLa in cycling, running and walking. *Scand J Rehab Med*, 9, pp. 69-77.

Bouchard, C. (2000). *Physical Activity and Obesity*. Human Kinetics, USA.

Brooks, D. and Brooks, C. (1995). *Stability Ball Programming Guide for Fitness Professionals*. Moves International Publishing, USA.

Brooks, D.S. (2004). *The Complete Book of Personal Training*. Human Kinetics, USA.

Brooks, G.A. (2000). *Exercise Physiology: Human Bioenergetics and Its Applications*. 3rd Ed. Mayfield Publications, USA.

Budget, R. (1990). Overturning syndrome. *British J Sports Med*, 24, pp. 231-236.

Burke, L. and Deakin V. (2000). *Clinical Sports Nutrition*. 2nd Ed. McGraw-Hill, USA.

Chia, M., Leong, L.L. and Quek, J.J. (2004). *Healthy, Well and Wise: Take PRIDE for a Life of Wellness*. National Institute of Education, Singapore.

Clarkson, P.M. and Nosaka, K. (1992). Muscle function after exercise – Induced muscle damage and rapid adaptation. *Med Sci Sports Exerc*, 24, pp. 512-520.

Daly, J. (2000). *Recreation and Sport Planning and Design*. 2nd Ed. Human Kinetics, USA.

Evans, W.J. (1995). Protein nutrition and resistance exercise. *Canadian J Appl Physiol*, 26 (Suppl), pp. S141-S152.

Fiala, K.A., Casa, D.J. and Roti, M.W. (2004). Rehydration with a caffeinated beverage during the non-exercise periods of 3 consecutive days of a 2-a-day practices. *Int J Sport Nutr Exerc Metabol*, 14, pp. 419-429.

Fitts, D.M. and Posner, M.I. (1967). *Human Performance*. Brooks/Cole, USA.

Fleck, S.J. (1988). Cardiovascular adaptations to resistance training. *Med Sci Sports Exerc*, 20(Suppl.), pp. S146-S151.

Gettman, L.R., et al. (1978). The effect of circuit weight training on strength, cardiorespiratory function and body composition of adult men. *Med Sci Sports Exerc*, 10, pp. 171-176.

Hardy, L. and Jones, D. (1986). Dynamic flexibility and proprioceptive neuromuscular facilitation. *Res Quarterly Exerc Sport*, 57, pp. 150-153.

Hawley, J.A. and Burke, L.M. (1997). Effect of meal frequency and timing on physical performance. *British J Nutr*, 77(Suppl), pp. S91-S103.

Haymes, E.M. (1991). Vitamin and mineral supplementation to athletes. *Int J Spt Nutr*, 1, pp. 146-169.

Heyward, V.H. (2002). *Advanced Fitness Assessment and Exercise Prescription*. 4th Ed. Human Kinetics, USA.

Howell, J.N. and Chleboun, G. (1993). Muscle stiffness, strength loss, swelling and soreness following exercise-induced injury to humans. *J Physiol*, 464, pp. 183-196.

Ivy, J.L., et al. (2002). Early post-exercise muscle glycogen recovery is enhanced with a carbohydrate-protein supplement. *J Appl Physiol*, 93, pp. 1337-1344.

Jackson, A.S. and Polluck, M.L. (1978). Generalised equations for predicting body density of men. *British J Nutr*, 40, pp. 497-504.

Jackson, A., et al. (1978). Intertester reliability of selected skinfold and circumference measurements and percent fat estimates. *Res Quarterly Exerc Sport*, 49, pp. 546-551.

Jackson, A., et al. (1980). Generalised equations for predicting body density of women. *Med Sci Sports Exerc*, 12, pp. 175-182.

Jequier, E. (1987). Energy, obesity and body weight standards. *Am J Clin Nutr*, 45, pp. 1035-1047.

Manninen, A.H. (2004). Protein hydrolysates in sports and exercise: A brief review. *J Sports Sci Med*, 3, pp. 60-63.

Mazzeo, R.S. (1998). ACSM position stand on exercise and physical activity for older adults. *Med Sci Sports Exerc*, 30, pp. 992-1008.

McArdle, W., et al. (2001). *Exercise Physiology: Energy, Nutrition, and Human Performance*. 5th Ed. Lippincott Williams & Wilkins, USA.

McAtee, R.E. and Charland, J. (1999). *Facilitated Stretching*. 2nd Ed. Human Kinetics, USA.

Olds, T. and Norton, K. (1996). *Anthropometrica: A Textbook of Body Measurements for Sports and Health Courses*. UNSW Press, Australia.

Prochaska, J.O., et al. (1992). In search of how people change: applications to addictive behaviours, *Am Psychol*, 47, pp. 1102–1114.

Rush, A.K. (1997). *The Modern Book of Stretching: Strength and Flexibility at Any Age*. Dell Publishing, New York.

Sullivan, M.G., et al. (1992). Effect of pelvic position and stretching method on hamstring muscle flexibility. *Med Sci Sports Exerc*, 24, pp. 1383-1389.

Tipton, K.D. and Wolfe, R.R. (2001). Exercise, protein metabolism, and muscle growth. *Int J Sports Nutr Exerc Metabol*, 11, pp. 109-132.

Waterhouse, J., et al. (2002). Identifying some determinants of 'jet lag' and its symptoms: A study of athletes and other travellers. *British J Sports Med*, 36, pp. 54-60.

Wolinsky, I. and Driskell, J.A. (2004). *Nutritional Ergogenic Aids*. CRC Press, USA.

Wong, P. and Lee, P.C. (2009) Managing obesity in Singapore schools – Holistic approaches for the future. In Aplin, N. (Ed) *Perspectives on Physical Education and Sports Science in Singapore – An Eye on the Youth Olympics 2010*. McGraw-Hill Education, Asia.

Zatsiorsky, V.M. (1995). *Science and Practice of Strength Training*. Human Kinetics, Champaign, IL.